DO MOTHERS DREAM OF ELECTRIC BABIES?

We live in a society that ignores and disregards attachment needs and feelings. Starting from this consideration, the author describes the stages of human emotional development in a lucid narrative which is both scientifically rigorous and grounded in clinical examples. Mieli critically investigates the origins of a specific weariness towards feelings which is reflected in the history of Western philosophy and science, resulting in a cultural disregard of emotional needs. The book powerfully suggests that if undeterred, this disregard may lead to severe consequences for the future of our society. Research compellingly shows that responding to fundamental emotional needs is a psycho-biological requirement necessary for human wellbeing and survival itself. Mieli contends that its oversight has a counterpart in the dramatic rise of mental distress in contemporary society, as well as in the difficulties that are increasingly encountered around maternity, fertility, and parenting.

Giuliana Mieli, PhD, DClinPsych, Psychotherapist, after working in the first mental health community services in the 1970s, has been a consultant in the maternity wards of St Gerardo Hospital (Monza) and at St Giuseppe Hospital (Milan) in Italy. Aside from clinical practice, she has dedicated herself to the psycho-education of medical and paramedical staff in various local health centres, and to training and supervising freshly graduated clinical psychologists and psycho-therapists. She is currently based in Florence.

DO MOTHERS DREAM OF ELECTRIC BABIES?

The Importance of Emotional Bonds for Growing, Nurturing, and Educating

Giuliana Mieli

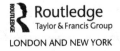

Routledge
Taylor & Francis Group

LONDON AND NEW YORK

First published in Italian in 2009 as
*Il bambino non è un elettrodomestico. Gli affetti che contano
per crescere, curare, educare*
by San Pablo Comunicacion SSP

First published 2019
by Routledge
2 Park Square, Milton Park, Abingdon, Oxon OX14 4RN

and by Routledge
711 Third Avenue, New York, NY 10017

Routledge is an imprint of the Taylor & Francis Group, an informa business

British Library Cataloguing-in-Publication Data
A catalogue record for this book is available from the British Library

Library of Congress Cataloging-in-Publication Data
A catalog record has been requested for this book

ISBN: 9-781-78220-353-7 (pbk)

CONTENTS

ACKNOWLEDGEMENT

I would like to thank my daughter, Lucia, for her help and support in making this English edition possible.

To Enzo Paci and Joseph Needham, who inspired me,
and to Costantino Mangioni, who let me learn by doing.

PREFACE

This book is not an academic essay: it is, rather, a journey through the emotional and professional experiences that, in my own life pathway, have brought me to understand what I will describe herein.

My intention in writing this book was to take the reader by the hand and accompany him or her through a process of experiencing and reasoning around birth which has fascinated and inspired me in the first place. No previous knowledge or expertise is required to read this book, as I did not aim to address a selective circle of specialised readers, but anyone who might share my interest around these themes. For this reason, in Chapters Three and Four, I chose not only to reference the authors who inspired me the most, but to quote their words in full so as to give the reader immediate access to texts which are otherwise difficult to get hold of, as most of them are no longer in circulation. Readers who have little or no interest in this theoretical part can simply skip it and move straight on to the next chapter.

For the sake of simplicity, in this book the child or baby of either gender will be generally referred to with masculine pronouns, unless otherwise specified. Since my aim has been to provide a meaning framework to our bio-psychological makeup, as designed in our evolutionary past, and explain how it gets expressed during the physiology of procreation supporting its felicitous outcome, in this book I will refer to "mother" and "father" as the primary and secondary caregivers; by this I mean two figures united to each other by a reciprocal choice of desire and made secure by a loving attachment bond which concretises in the wish for a child. Obviously, in the course of history as well as today, other emotionally bonded figures have come to effectively impersonate the roles of the caregiving couple, but I believe that knowing what nature prepared for in terms of bio-psychological needs and their organisation remains fundamental for all good caregiving.

INTRODUCTION

"Elderly primiparous ..." was the startling expression that inaugurated my journey as a pregnant thirty-nine-year-old when I first sought the services of a maternity ward. I vividly remember how this blunt statement profoundly shocked me at the time. It immediately triggered an intense feeling of shame, as if someone were standing there scolding me for having waited too long—something that, however unpleasant, I was willing to accept—but also suggesting that this delay could have less than positive or even adverse effects on the outcome of my pregnancy. I felt stricken, as I said, by those words, just as I would be in so many instances and procedures I was going to be subjected to during my gestation: just to name the most invasive one, an amniocentesis test[1] that was unrequested and performed on me without prior information. This feeling of uncertainty, helplessness, intrusion, and shame would accompany me in all my pregnancies. Then, all I could do was just bear it, whereas only much later I would learn to consider it and understand its roots in a different light. Later, when the circumstances of life led me to my transformation from a psychotherapist working in pioneering psychiatry to an "expert" in motherhood.

But let us take a step back. My first university degree was not in psychotherapy, but in theoretical philosophy. This was a subject that had fascinated me since high school but which I had had to drop until the events of 1968 gave access to the humanities to students who had majored in scientific studies in the lower grades. In fact, I had also been passionate about physics and chemistry, so much so that my graduate thesis, eventually, ended up being a comparative analysis between Western and Chinese developments in philosophical and scientific thought. I was tutored through this difficult but fascinating research by the unforgettable Enzo Paci, and it was he who directed me to the writings of Joseph Needham.

An embryologist and biologist, Needham had been a leading figure in Cambridge since the 1930s, a time when prominent physicists like Rutherford, Bohr, and Heisenberg were intent on grappling with the recent discoveries in physics. At the turn of the century, the momentous introduction of groundbreaking theories such as Einstein's relativity, quantum theory, the particle-wave theory of light, and the uncertainty principle (just to name a few) had, in fact, fundamentally challenged the basic theories at the roots of classic Western science. Years later, Needham confided to me how the climate in Cambridge back then was one of restless excitement and fierce debating. He was, therefore, surprised to notice that the reaction of the Chinese exchange students in physics and chemistry was, instead, strikingly at odds with the general mood. In particular, they appeared little shaken by the observation of the dual nature of matter and of its dynamism, a concept that, far from clashing with Chinese ancient philosophy, they told him fitted perfectly with it. Needham was fascinated by this revelation, and went on to become the greatest sinologist of the twentieth century. My encounter with him allowed me to understand, through another culture's philosophy, the advantages and limitations of "classical scientific thought", which I came to discover was not a transparent outlook on nature. Instead, I learnt to read it as a relative and historically construed framework grounded in determinism and mechanism. In the Western world, however, this approach continues to prevail as *the* rational point of view to the understanding of nature, serving up false, shortsighted certainties wherever applied to realms of enquiry whose complexity exceeds its heuristic power.

My studies in philosophy and comparative sciences allowed me instead to develop a capacity, or, rather, naturalness, which I later brought to my work as a therapist, to stay with things, resisting the urge to classify, following the very contemporary (and very Chinese) belief in the continual transformative power of life and energy. These studies also provided me with the assurance that seemingly unknown or strange clusters of phenomena can, in a context capable of understanding, transform themselves and be resolved.

But I would not stop there, in the world of academia. More than in speculation, I was, in fact, interested in action. I wanted to find a way, a field where my speculative passion—which had led me to break out of the invisible rules guiding that flat, "normal" reasoning which had proved incapable of grasping the complexity of life, the unity of matter–energy, the complete correspondence of body and mind—could find active expression and become a way towards change.

Therefore, I turned my attention to social research and, fascinated and enthused by my meeting with Giulio Maccacaro,[2] took part in the first mental health centres opened countrywide just before the Basaglia reform abolished mental asylums in Italy. I had to get a second degree, one in Clinical Psychology, to be allowed to work as a psychotherapist, but it was well worth the effort. Field experience with seriously ill patients, both in hospitals and elsewhere around the country, confirmed to me that the distress expressed in "folly" actually had, rather than organic, deep emotional origins, which were rooted in each individual's history and had been reinforced by social and cultural double-binds.

My experience with psychiatric patients powerfully conveyed to me how human beings, in order to survive and actualise their creative potential, need not only food and shelter, but also love. This is when I also discovered that the expression of love cannot be *haphazard*, but that there is an innate, biological template governing the arousal and expression of feelings, which stands at the root of our survival and well-being. I discovered, in fact, that this template is not only useful, but also *necessary* for the survival of the species. If altered, distorted, or abused by the socioeconomic power dynamics or by cultural values—be it in the life of an individual or in society as a whole—the penalty is dramatic: suffering, pain, distress, and, ultimately, madness as a last defence of the self, stating the impossibility of survival as a human being under those circumstances, as well as upheavals, decay, and the risk of the dissolution of society on a greater scale.

Working in the first community mental health centres, at the forefront of the struggle for the recognition of the social origins of mental health diseases, was, therefore, an intense and enriching experience for me. However, as I became pregnant and with the birth of my own children, I found that I did not have it in me to pursue this full-time work further. Trusting my emotions as meaningful and protecting what is important for well-being, I actually determined that I would not give up the joy of looking after my children. Therefore, I set up a small private practice, and held back my nostalgia for the socially engaged work I did at the mental health centres for the time being.

It was a hospital—St Gerardo, in Monza—that opened the door for me to return to work within the public sector, the same hospital I stumbled into when, as an "elderly primiparous", I was desperately seeking a more humane, caring environment than the one I had encountered at other maternity services. A more humane environment that I did find at St Gerardo, where, after coming to know me and my previous work, I was asked by the Head Physician if I would be interested in helping to set up the prenatal courses.

So it was that, pregnant among pregnant women, I began observing obstetricians and doctors at work. I started to study and learn, and to apply my philosophical speculations and experience as a psychotherapist to a completely new field for me, the field of motherhood.

Notes

1. A procedure in which, around the fourth month of pregnancy, a sample of amniotic fluid is drawn through the mother's abdomen to extract cells of foetal origin, for the purpose of DNA screening for genetic abnormalities. The test can be risky for the mother and foetus and nowadays it is compulsory to obtain informed consent to perform it.
2. A doctor, biologist and statistician who became a prominent figure in sociological and epidemiological research applied to mental health in the 1970s in Italy.

CHAPTER ONE

My clinical experience in a maternity ward

Mixed in among pregnant women, an anonymous observer in the pregnant public attending the prenatal courses, I first of all noted how a great deal of *information* was being given regarding birth and the post-partum period.

For instance, techniques were taught regarding breathing and relaxation, and a great emphasis was also placed on the importance of breastfeeding. However, none of this I found was in any way justified or backed up by an explanation of the intrinsic link between human subjective experience, as expressed in our emotions, and its embodied manifestation in the body. I noticed with amazement that no mention was made of the extraordinary physical and emotional transformations we each undergo, as children, during our slow development along the demanding, gradual pathway from symbiosis to separation through the difficult conquest of autonomy. In other words, it seemed to me that rules of hygiene and behaviour were being recommended without any grounding within a meaningful framework based on a proper philosophical or psychological understanding of human nature.

How and *what* were covered, but not *why*. The result was that the courses conveyed a set of overall superficial instructions, which I sensed would be easily uprooted by any pseudo-information or fad that parents might eventually come to contact with via all sorts of dubious means of communication, as happens with increasing frequency in our culture. The outcome I observed was a noticeable anxiety among the pregnant women, all sincerely wishing to be adequately prepared for motherhood and all genuinely interested in learning how to act in order to be most useful to their children. However, instead of a framework capable of providing them with authentic guidance, they were instead showered with loads of information and over-detailed, contrasting directions that were, overall, both insufficiently explanatory and contradictory, which easily created disorientation.

For someone like me, accustomed as I was through the practice of psychotherapy to restoring disturbed emotional balances and to healing the emotional debris left by damaging child-rearing practices suffered early in life by my adult clients, it seemed shocking to see that, in a place like this, where children were brought into life, no serious guidance was given in the courses as to what constitutes emotionally healthy parenting. No mention was made of the importance of respecting, understanding, and supporting the child's needs and growth, and of safeguarding both his physical *and* his emotional well-being. No information whatsoever was provided to increase awareness in mothers and fathers as to what child development entails and what role they would soon be called upon to play to facilitate it. The prenatal courses did not, in particular, provide vital information as to how the child's slow process of emancipation from dependence to emotional autonomy is, in fact, dependent on the consistent and secure presence and support of *qualitatively specific* parental templates of responses to the baby's irreducible developmental needs.

I spoke to doctors and midwives in the ward about this bewildering omission in the courses but, to my even greater surprise, I realised they appeared completely oblivious as to the point I was trying to make. I was dumbstruck. Although I did not expect them to be informed about the latest discoveries in evolutionary psychology, I had taken for granted a minimum knowledge of how emotions are organised in relation to the interpersonal context that evokes them: some intuitive common sense, at the very least an experiential awareness of the instinctive set of emotions inevitably evoked in doctor–patient relationships. Even here, in fact, there is a "little one" and a "grown-up": one in need who yields, entrusting herself to the other's care, and a more knowledgeable other who is called upon to meet this trust and attend to the patient's needs.

I was surprised because ignorance of this fact is not only likely to generate disastrous misunderstandings in doctor–patient communication (just as the same ignorance creates disasters in parenting relationships), but also because not knowing about the basic emotional dynamic underlying caring relationships prevents doctors from being able to do their job effectively and efficiently. Their care, in fact, would require less effort if they knew how to embody and deploy a specific pattern of relating intrinsic to any caring role. I am referring to that qualitatively salient attitude of emotional availability and non-judgemental openness to listen, which is especially apt to hold and contain latencies, uncertainty, anxieties, questions, and doubts which the patient naturally bestows upon her doctor, seeking a soothing response. If the doctor keeps his distance and communication is cold and impersonal, the message actually conveyed to the one in need is not neutral, but, rather, transmits that the emotionality of the doctor–patient relation is rejected, with the consequence that this unaddressed emotional tension could have a negative impact on the outcome of care.

Why on earth were my colleagues unaware of the importance of the relational aspect of their care? Were they aware that their patients were persons? Did they have an adequate enough concept of "person" to be able to relate to one? I came to understand that today's medicine focuses on the sickness, not the patient. "Elderly primiparous" was beginning to sound like the sign of a certain mentality: the result of a school of thought that transforms patients from persons to a constellation of symptoms on which a set protocol of interventions is performed.

Compared to the doctors, the nurses and midwives on the maternity ward were less distant and more emotionally participant (though not always appropriately). The relationship itself with the patient was closer and longer, as well as more direct, with a subtler definition of roles and less interference from technology. There was more room for familiarity and spontaneity, allowing for a more integrated perception of the patient's needs, expectations, anxieties, doubts, and fears.

On the other hand, doctors looked more like "unwitting parents" with regard to their patients' needs: shrouded in their white coats, stethoscopes hanging around their necks, they appeared indifferent to, or even disturbed by, the anxious expectations of their patients.

These, in turn, appeared shrunken during interactions with the medical staff, as if reduced to fragile human beings facing disagreeable, inscrutable deities. I was, however, to discover that this aseptic approach was not considered problematic, but, on the contrary, the prerequisite of an effective doctor–patient relationship. Medical schools, in fact, actually recommend and teach this attitude as the standard, the only means to control and prevent—in doctor and patient alike—an otherwise dangerous, disturbing, and unscientific emotional involvement from forming.

As I reflected on all this, a new opportunity for an exchange with the medical staff came my way. I was asked to take charge of delivering prenatal diagnoses, which, in this context, refers to the outcome of early tests carried out to identify any foetal anomalies. This obviously involved dealing with feelings of pain, risk, and failure, feelings that we might not like, but which are inherent emotional components of childbirth just as much as are desire, expectant trepidation, and hope. They are much more "inconvenient" to hold, however, since they directly correlate to loss and inadequacy: to a defeat of the project, to a failure of the caring environment. Even in the doctors' perspective, in these instances an aseptic attitude was no longer fruitful, but it was recognised as an inadequate tool for dealing with pain. Suddenly, emotions, which had been thrown out of the window as unscientific and dangerous confounding variables by the medical diktat, were now coming back through the door; the request was for me, a "psychologist", to become a sort of "bereavement expert" and be left to deal with all these inconvenient feelings they wanted nothing to do with.

Naturally, I refused to play this role. I felt, in fact, that accepting the management of the problematic cases would have meant being collusive with the general denial of affectivity in place among the medical staff. If I had complied, I felt I would have confirmed, and even implicitly authorised, the prevailing schism between the purely medical and the emotional aspects of care. It would have meant abiding with the notion that the emotional aspect of childbirth ought to be taken care of only when absolutely necessary: namely at times of bereavement and suffering linked to failure.

Since then, I have taken it upon myself to spread awareness of the scientific fact that there is no life without the affective process that underpins our experience of being alive; we simply cannot cleanse it out, and neither should we. Our emotional experience of events is, in fact, comparable to our physical perception of hot and cold, hunger, thirst, or tiredness; it provides human beings with a fundamental sixth sense fostering the survival of our species. In the same way as physical perceptions, our feelings provide us with the basis to identify whether any given context, be it physical or interpersonal, fosters our well-being or hinders it. If recognised and listened to, our feelings, therefore, guide us towards addressing what causes us pain or distress, promoting well-being through the active negotiation of a better relationship with the environment, both physical and interpersonal. Fear, anger, joy, curiosity, trust, suspicion, anxiety, pleasure, desire, sympathy, and so many other emotions explain to us our environment and what surrounds us. Nothing happens in a vacuum. There is always some kind of feeling to go with our living body and this ends only with our physical death. It is never really possible to be unaffected by the feelings that we feel and by the ones experienced by the people who surround us.

Accordingly, I did not like the idea that only when dealing with bereavement should we suddenly notice the emotional component that permeates pregnancy. I could not accept the notion that pregnancy and childbirth might be reduced to purely physical events, shunning the myriad feelings that accompany and orientate us through this process. I felt that the emotional component had to be reconsidered and reaffirmed so that, at least at the moment of birth, life could be restored to its complexity, poetry, and to its mystery and sacredness.

Therefore, instead of accepting the bereavement expert role, I proposed that the doctors joined me in a "training in affectivity". In the course of our encounters, I would provide them with an understanding of the meaning, function, and organisation of emotions, something that would help them to acknowledge, regulate, and deal with their own emotions as well as those of their patients, making them aware of how crucial a role they play in accompanying women through the adventure of childbirth. This would accustom them to navigating and dealing with their own limitations, with pain and failure, all inevitable parts of their lives and profession, with no magical cures or escapes, but manageable only through empathy, participation, sharing, and solidarity.

*   *   *

I will never forget a significant episode I witnessed in the obstetrics A&E, which happened at around that time. In preparation for the training, I was given the task of observing doctor–patient relationships during consultations so as to be able to point out and eventually work through any deficiencies in emotional communication I might identify. Consequently, in my white coat and without revealing my true identity, for a while I stationed myself in the obstetric visiting centre, observing in complete silence and withholding any comment for a later moment.

One day, I entered a consulting room just as a young doctor was seeing a couple of more or less her own age. The woman had suffered some bleeding and the doctor was trying to explain to the couple how it was impossible, given the early stage of the young woman's pregnancy, to make a proper diagnosis of what was happening simply on the basis of an ultrasound scan. That meant that there was no way of knowing whether or not the patient was still pregnant, or if she had had a miscarriage, or if her pregnancy was extra-uterine. The patient was to go home and not be left alone, just in case there was any more haemorrhaging.

With every new hypothesis regarding her condition, I saw the patient—a slim, emaciated young woman with a pained look—sink deeper into her seat, curling up as if to protect herself from the increasingly painful darts with which she was being bombarded. She looked terrified and helpless, while the doctor coolly rattled off the various medical hypotheses and not one word more. This was July and it was very hot. The patient's companion, who was standing beside her, was wearing only an undershirt, barely concealing what once might have been a handsome body but which had now grown stout. Nevertheless, he had a manly "leave it to me" attitude, taking in every diagnosis in the way in which one would parry a blow and showing an incredible ability to think positively. He would be the one to look after her at home; he would even take time off work. From the way he spoke, you could tell this was not the first time they had tried to have a child, hitherto unsuccessfully. But this time, whatever the outcome might be, at least she was pregnant, which meant that his own undergoing of an operation for a varicocele on his scrotum—a varicose enlargement of the veins of the spermatic cord—had been useful. While the couple sadly walked out of the room, I felt pity for that quiet, emaciated-looking young woman who was dying of shame and guilt for still not having made it to motherhood.

I was still thinking back on the sad episode and weighing the options of suggesting to the doctor a slightly more participative and concerned approach with her patients, when, all of a sudden, the consulting room was invaded by an exuberant gypsy. I suddenly remembered having seen her outside as she paced up and down the waiting area. She was a young and breathtakingly beautiful woman, with a cheerful face lit up by a pair of bright green eyes, and she was obviously pregnant, with her belly jutting out boldly. Not in the slightest bit shy, she came in without knocking and came to a halt in the middle of the room. She demanded a scan: she wanted to see her baby. No, she did not have an appointment, and neither did she want to make one; she could not wait; she was a ride operator with an itinerant funfair and who knew where she would be tomorrow with her caravan? "Quick, doctor, show me my baby!" The young doctor was taken aback by such determined assertiveness. She tried to appeal again to the need for an appointment, but to no avail. In the end, having tried in every way to put her off, she gave in and, against all rules and regulations, proceeded to see the patient, throwing desperate glances in my direction in search of some complicity from me.

The gypsy answered evasively to the usual basic questions; she was vague about the number of children she already had, and even more vague about when she had had her last period. As she was getting ready, shedding layer upon layer of colourful skirts to take her place for the examination behind the screen "so I can see my baby", a more experienced male doctor who had previously been called in for a consultation on the previous patient's case, unexpectedly walked into the room. He was an old acquaintance of mine, happy to see me, and asked what I was doing there. Before I had time to answer, the gypsy woman instantly jumped up, grabbed my male colleague by the shoulders and shouting "A man!" literally threw him out of the room without any of us daring to intervene. So it was that she finished her examination undisturbed and far from what her culture had obviously made her experience as male prying eyes.

I remember feeling at that moment as if the gypsy's healthy impetuosity, her guileless, direct defence of her needs, redressed the scales somewhat towards avenging the shy little frightened patient who came before her. The young doctor, who had managed the earlier patient in strict accordance with medical school recommendations, had clearly suffered a destabilising blow to her hard-won aseptic stance; a blow brought to her by a simple, probably ignorant person who merely clung tenaciously to her powerful, explosive, emotional need to "see her baby", not taking no for an answer.

CHAPTER TWO

From undifferentiated to differentiated. Birth, growth, and the achievement of independence: an emotional perspective

I n the human animal, pregnancy lasts forty weeks. This is, arguably, a very long time, but it is so designed to protect and foster what needs to be a slow and delicate process. Similarly, the child's process of separation from parental figures after birth needs to be a slow and gradual one. The need for this becomes apparent if we just think of the complexity of the neurological and emotional development that needs to take place within the facilitative environment represented by the relationship with our carers. Nowadays, the World Health Organization sets the age that marks adult autonomy at twenty-four.

In considering this slow process of emancipation from infantile dependence to adult autonomy, I find we often forget to take into full account its deeper meaning. There is, in fact, a difficult and complex process that must take place within the primary relationships so that a sense of security—a *sine qua non* condition for survival, let alone well-being—can transform from being dependent on the contingent availability of unconditional support, originally ensured through the physical and emotional symbiosis with mother, to gradually become a feature of emotional autonomy of the self. This is what, in turn, makes it possible for adult human beings to navigate the world, to plan and make responsible choices.

This transformation of security from an interpersonal to an autonomous feature takes place by way of the slow internalisation of the dependability of the earliest experiences of care through their repetition and gradual modification over time to accommodate the child's expanding capacities. In their watchful and attuned participation, parents, hormonally and emotionally equipped for this role, fulfil their core task when they support and facilitate the passage from security in dependence to autonomous self-confidence for their children.

Compared to other animals, human beings are equipped with a far greater capacity for self-determination, agency, and for changing the environment to accommodate their needs, rather than adapt to the *status quo*. Nevertheless, we are conditioned in our ability and freedom by a physical and emotional physiology pertaining to our nature as animal-men. This dictates clear, unavoidable conditions for our survival, for our well-being, and for attaining an emotional quality of existence which is more fundamental than usually supposed.

Following his free will, in fact, a man can easily drink cyanide or jump from the tenth floor of a building. However, having disobeyed the natural rules of physical survival, he would not live to tell of his expression of "free choice". Our considerable freedom is, therefore, *not unconditional*, but unavoidably linked to the natural laws of an environment in which we live and from which human beings cannot escape. Before addressing mental distress, psychology is—or should be—the science that studies the emotional and relational conditions that allow our survival and well-being. If we did not know them, or they did not exist, in fact, how could we claim we could help our clients restore them and feel better?

In the history of Western thought, it has never been sufficiently considered or scientifically theorised that human survival is not only dependent on certain physical requirements, but that emotional conditions also exist and are just as binding. The discovery and scientific theorisation of these binding emotional conditions for human existence is only recent and seem not to have been translated into common knowledge or to have made an impact on the organisation of our social life yet. This ignorance represents, I would argue, a severe danger for our survival, at least as much as the blind form of technological development that is currently threatening the preservation of life on earth. On the contrary, I believe that the introduction of a cultural perspective capable of considering human beings in all their inconvenient yet splendid complexity—a perspective, therefore, able to make us aware of the conditions which are necessary for the full realisation of our humanity—could inspire a revolution in thought. I am not alone in this awareness. As a society, we are, in fact, becoming more and more aware of a need for a cultural shift to embrace a meaningful framework for life based on a more attentive consideration of the quality of relationships. A framework, therefore, centred on, and capable of, creating the *specific* conditions which foster human well-being within nature, is the only possible way forward if we want to overcome the current crisis our society is facing.

> When Teilhard de Chardin predicted, fifty years ago, that humans would one day learn how to harness the energies of love and that such a development would be as pivotal in the history of mankind as the discovery of fire, his vision was regarded as purely utopian. Not so today, for in the closing decades of the twentieth century the nature of love and how the capacity to love develops has become a subject for scientific study, the implications of which are at least as important as those of genetics, electronics or the quantum theory. (Odent, 1999, p. 1)

The emotional experience of pregnancy: mother, father, and child

In order to understand the physiological organisation of emotions underlying secure attachment bonds, it could be argued that there is nothing more eloquent than looking at the origin of human life, letting it speak to us emotionally as well as rationally. In human beings, we find, in fact, a close link between physical and emotional development, provided this synchronicity is facilitated rather than hindered. By this, I mean that the stages of physical and emotional maturation are meant to coincide, but the two aspects can run smoothly parallel only if their distinctive meanings and mutual interdependence are taken into account.

Human beings begin their adventure in life emerging from symbiosis. We begin our lives *thanks to* a relationship—from the standpoint of evolution, the loving encounter between a man and a woman—and *within* a very close relationship: the one between the maternal body and the embryo, which implies an emotional and corporeal fusion, a symbiosis.

If I dwell upon the nature and quality of this beginning, it is because it is difficult to understand the emotional journey made by human beings during their existence unless we carefully consider where it all starts. Insightfully, some Eastern cultures set the beginning of an individual's existence not at delivery, but at conception, so that the nine months inside the mother's womb are counted in. This tradition embodies an ancient philosophical wisdom which understood the importance of the prenatal period not so much for the physical development that takes place in the uterus, but essentially because its consideration facilitates an understanding of human beings in our more complex essence as psycho-physical units. To rephrase, the prenatal period is an important part of development just as any other, but it becomes an essential one to consider in order to understand how and why it unfolds as it does. From the moment the egg and the sperm cell meet, it is in the uterus that we find not only the prelude to, and foundations of, physical development, but also the beginning of an emotional and sensory perception of being alive that, just like the body, precedes the moment of birth.

What the mother feels

It is common wisdom that, at the beginning of human life, lies the encounter between egg and sperm, adult sexual cells from physically and, one hopes, emotionally mature individuals. We shall find, however, that, contrary to popular belief, although necessary, this condition is in itself not sufficient for a baby to be born.

I once watched a fascinating video that showed the fertilised egg descend along the Fallopian tube, dancing lightly like a multi-coloured soap bubble not yet subject to gravity, until reaching the walls of the uterus. There, thanks to the thickening of the endometrium (the mucus membrane coating the walls of the uterus) provoked by a specific hormonal change aimed at facilitating implantation, the egg could nest within the wall's villosity and, through this sudden contact, the cell would begin to grow.

Let us take a moment to consider this. It is the rekindling of a connection—again a symbiosis—and not mere fertilisation that gives the go-ahead for life: the fertilised egg must be nested in a welcoming endometrium prepared by hormonal modification, otherwise it will simply slip away and be lost.

We can gather from this observation how nature suggests, from the very beginning, that for the purpose of survival, human life needs a welcoming environment, that is, one suitable for life to express itself. Any premature interruption of this early connection between baby and mother-environment, whether caused by physical or emotional factors, will lead to risks to the pregnancy or even failure, as we shall see.

Following this insight, which shows that the woman needs to become a facilitative and nurturing environment from the moment of fertilisation and not just from birth onwards, we may observe that nature works on the expectant mother and on her body through changes that *already* favour an increased attitude towards nursing. The physical and emotional modifications that occur during pregnancy are, in sum, not cursory epiphenomena, but important signals for the woman to experience and understand. Once properly deciphered, in fact, they can give meaningful suggestions as to the right attitude the woman will need to actively bring to her nursing and mother role once the baby is born. In this light, pregnancy and childbirth are truly extraordinary events, capable of inspiring a profound reflection on the physical and emotional needs of human life: a real treatise on psychology in a nutshell and an invaluable head start for any philosophical enquiry aiming to gain an insight into the meaning of human life.

Nature first expresses the templates of care and concern for new life within and through the body and emotions of the mother, because that is where the child is formed. We must then read what happens and take it into account if we want to seize and understand the message that is buried within this covert—in the sense of out of sight—process.

But let us take a step back. Males and females differ not only physically but also hormonally, hence in how they emotionally process and experience the world. Indeed, if we consider the survival of our species when we evolved, males and females have been clearly designed to perform complementary functions. During adolescence, males reach a hormonal peak that more or less remains constant over time. Their bodies become more robust. Nature equips them physically and emotionally to fulfil their role in the physical fight for survival. It seems self-evident, when men first came out of their primitive cave dwellings, if they had had the same physical and emotional endowment as women, the human race would have probably become extinct long ago.

Women, on the other hand, entrusted as they are with the tasks of conceiving and nursing the offspring, are endowed with a more vulnerable physical makeup, yet one marked by an enhanced flexibility and finer perceptive sensitivity. The core of the maternal role lies in the capacity to attune to, and mould oneself to meet the child's needs. In contrast to the relative hormonal stability of males, the mature female endocrinological makeup follows a cyclical pattern, reaching a peak and then declining on a monthly basis. This makes women more sensitive and emotionally flexible, a feature designed to help them perform the psychologically complex role of shifting between their own adult experience of the world while also being able to identify with that of their child and to his emotional needs in order to meet them. Sensitive women, even in the absence of an offspring, can, in fact, feel their mood markedly change at the time of ovulation and menstruation, respectively the creative peak and the moment of decline within the monthly fertility cycle.

Conception is, therefore, a meeting of two worlds: the male and the female one, which we could think of as two complementary, but not overlapping, domains. They can be intended as two emotional fields from the perspective of which men and women inherently explore and interpret reality, which becomes integrated in the forming of the parenting couple, thus setting the stage of the experiential world within which the newborn will securely move.

In is important to note, however, that male and female emotional fields do not equal man and woman. Men have a small share of female hormones, just as women have a small share of male hormones, allowing for a partial overlap in each individual of the two emotional fields and ensuing experience of the world. This facilitates mutual understanding and perspective taking between the genders as well as the negotiation of tasks and roles within the couple and society at large (or, at least, it should).

During pregnancy, a woman is subjected to important hormonal changes. A sensitive woman, or one who has already had a child, has no need for a pregnancy test to know she is expecting. She can tell. Nature actually sends signals in this sense that cannot be missed: nausea, squeamishness, sleepiness, and fatigue, all transformations of a woman's usual experience that convey that something has happened. This occurs mostly during the first three months of pregnancy, at a stage when there are not any marked physical changes that could reveal the early pregnancy. A pregnant woman should, all the more then, be able to listen to herself and yield to these new feelings: reducing physical exertion for instance, but also indulging her sense of fatigue and a sort of new inclination towards absorption in her internal world which often marks the beginning of this great adventure.

If she has a job, it would be a thousand times more logical for her to be protected from heavy or stressful work at the beginning of her pregnancy instead of during the last three months, when the size of her body would in any case prevent her involvement in excessively exertive tasks. Miscarriages during the first twelve weeks, on the other hand, are very frequent, so much so that many doctors consider them to be almost physiological.

We could, then, interpret the uneasiness of the first months as nature sending its message to the woman by way of physical and emotional signals, alerting her that something important is happening and suggesting she takes good care of herself and of the process taking place inside her. Women accustomed to paying attention to their dreams—which carry meaningful information about what is happening in our existences expressed in a language different from the one of waking life, unfettered by the rules of space and time, cause and effect—can also detect in these clear signs of ovulation and implantation, as well as of miscarriage and loss when things go wrong.

Uterine symbiosis is never, in fact, a purely physical event. It is only we Westerners who tend to read it that way. In humans, the emotional is always inherently interdependent with the physical, and cannot be otherwise. When a woman becomes pregnant, her hormonal cycle is modified by an increase in progesterone. This, you will remember, is the hormone responsible for thickening the endometrium, thereby guaranteeing and protecting the encounter between the fertilised egg and the womb, that is, the physical connection between mother and baby at the origin of life. But the symbiotic meeting facilitated and protected by this hormonal modification does not relate to the body only. It also has, contextually and just as importantly, an emotional counterpart. I refer here to that well-known alteration of a woman's mood that occurs during gestation, that often-mocked fiery heightening of feminine sensibility, clearly linked with the new hormonal state. But it seems no one has ever asked *why* nature has programmed this apparently uncontrolled explosion of the woman's feelings in pregnancy. This modification is, in fact, not a chance event (as rarely in biology there are such), but, rather, something that serves a purpose: serving the survival of the species.

This overpowering bursting of emotions, which erodes the space for rationality and often exposes forgotten memories, takes the woman back to that preverbal experience of the world pertaining to infancy where emotional perception alone works as means of assessing and reacting to the environment. We could say that what happens to the woman on the emotional level is somehow comparable to what happens to her physically. Gaining weight in her belly, a woman gradually loses her centre of gravity and, from her erect state, she is prompted to "fall" into the child's orbit: to take her baby's perspective. It is an identification that will allow the future mother—from any latitude, ethnicity, class, or culture—to guess and contingently respond to her child's needs expressed in an a-specific simple cry, made binding by the baby's vulnerability and inexperience.

For many women, this return to the past, this step back into childhood, can be a difficult experience. It often involves facing strong emotions and forgotten ways of feeling that are hard to regulate. It is like suddenly finding oneself as an infant, unable to handle or contain the movements of the soul. It is like looking at the world through the eyes of a baby, putting adult self-confidence aside, and reliving out the conditions of one's childhood, as it actually has been for each of us.

Considering the woman's shift in sensibility in this light represents an essential element to understand not only the physiological roots, but also many of the emotional and physical complications that may arise during gestation.

Pregnancy, by its very nature, is a state of *passive* symbiosis: during those nine long months, a woman cannot act upon her baby, and neither can she voluntarily and actively participate in his development. She can only adapt to the change and transformation that takes place in herself, body and mind, and it is best if she does so knowingly and serenely.

Many women describe pregnancy as a totally blissful state; other women experience discomforts of varying severity, such as nausea in the first trimester, stomach problems, insomnia, swelling in the legs, haemorrhoids, and constipation.

This is because babies do not develop inside the womb like pudding filling a mould. On the contrary, it is the maternal container that makes space, gradually swelling and yielding to wrap around the shape of the growing foetus. I like to think that what goes on inside the womb can be seen as an embodiment of the very kernel of maternal love. This is, in fact, a love that, emotionally too, contains the infant in a space that is first physical, then mental, allowing for the child's free and spontaneous movement within boundaries meant to keep him secure, but not constricted. It is the mother who adapts to her child, not the other way round. She is the one who makes room for the baby by the swelling of her womb and compression of her organs (stomach, intestines, and bladder) to hold him more comfortably.

The hidden lesson embodied in the process is, thus, that maternal means holding but not compressing. A child must occupy a space that is both physical and mental, which has to be irreducible. This will be the same after birth as well; the mother will initially have to give up much (if not all) of her space and time, to then become able to regain her autonomy and freedom only very slowly. In physiology, this "self-less" process is, however, designed to be time-limited and marked by extraordinary pleasure, supported by the very special emotional modification that comes with maternity.

It is difficult to describe the emotions of a woman who has been trying for a baby when she finally discovers she is pregnant. During the first three months, the child's presence is only something sensed, perceived through your body's alterations and sometimes through a mild unease that prevents you from carrying on living as before, forcing you into different rhythms, facilitating meditation and rest. This perception is even more conspicuous in our contemporary world, where everybody is constantly in a state of hectic productivity and where inactivity usually coincides with the end of one's strength: an enforced rest.

But if a mother-to-be lets herself indulge these physical and emotional sensations, what starts is a process of recovering an ancient way of relating to the self and the world; a mode of experiencing whereby the flow of one's feelings can be felt without forcing them to be different from what they are, and where the sense of time and life assumes another rhythm and another meaning. The habit of unconsciously adhering to a style of experiencing and behaving which is standardised and shared within our culture is substituted by a stance of mindful opening, listening, experiencing which adheres to a more natural way of life, marked by letting things happen, where doing becomes harmonious with being. The mother-to-be is invited to return to a childhood dimension where things have meaning and pleasure "here and now", where time accompanies existence rather than squeezing it in an urgent rush.

Towards the end of the fourth month, the feel of the first twitch, the quickening that signals the baby's live and complicit presence, engulfs the mother in a state of mysterious entrancement. The blissful intimacy of being two in one, the certainty of a constant presence which appeases, in the mother too, that universal longing for a sense of connection capable of soothing the fatigue and solitude of human life. For a woman who lets herself experience her feelings, pregnancy can be a bit of a dreamlike, "delirious" state; as if the rules of life were momentarily suspended and the never-lost dream of omnipotence could be true for a fraction of a second.

It is only the discomforts of pregnancy, the bulk and weight towards the end, the difficulty with movement and shortness of breath that gradually encourages and justifies the wish and desire for a different form of meeting. In fact, even in physiological pregnancies, some form of discomfort always emerges, if only for the progressive swelling and heaviness of the belly, which inevitably becomes more and more cumbersome with the passing of time. Very wisely, we could say, nature—while still protecting the fusional state and profound enjoyment of gestation—has added some elements of discomfort that tarnish the mother's creative omnipotence, the excessive perfection of completeness, in order to emotionally prepare her for the separation. Even in the utter bliss of pregnancy, after a time, in fact, the presence of some difficulty encourages the wish for another kind of connection with the child to arise. A certain discomfort also conveys the message that nothing, however much desired, can be achieved without patience and effort: an important reminder of the commitment that looking after a baby and meeting his needs will demand.

What the baby feels

To try to understand the experience of a foetus in the womb, we need to consider that a human body, from the moment it starts to develop, is never a mere body, but a body that "feels". When I say "feels", and I put this in inverted commas, I mean more than just physical perception, which surely is partly, but not fully, responsible for the more complex "feeling" to which I refer here. I am, in fact, more broadly alluding to the body's somatosensory appraisal of a state of either overall well-being or malaise. This, we find, in all higher animals but particularly in humans, depends not only and not so much on the satisfaction of our physical needs, but is instead strongly dependent on the more or less harmonious relationship the individual finds with the surrounding environment. And it is precisely in this relationship with an environment capable of meeting the physical and emotional needs that pertain to our nature that, from the beginning and through the entire course of our lives, the possibility for happiness lies.

Right after birth and not only inside the womb, the first environment we encounter is again not just a physical one, but it is, first and foremost, identified with the person who responds to (attunes to, understands, contains, and satisfies) the baby's primary physical needs. Ideally, this provision shadows the very same meeting of the infant's basic needs which used to happen automatically within the womb. In the English language, this is what truly underlies the word *care*: a quality of looking after that is attentive, thoughtful, generous, and selfless. *Caring*, in this sense, accompanies the satisfaction of physical and emotional needs and gives a feeling of well-being. No living creature exists that cannot appraise whether the quality of the surrounding environment is good or bad. In this sense, the transition from childhood to adulthood is a transition from "feeling" without being able to do anything—except benefit from a good fit or adapt to suffering—to "feeling" and eventually being capable of acting to change things.

Inside the womb, the somatosensory perception of well-being is essentially physical. But this does not mean that the picture is not wholly registered and internalised into an embodied "feel", even if not exactly mentalized. I often compare life in the womb with the idea that, within our culture, we have construed of paradise. The uterus is, in effect, a place perfectly adapted to meet the baby's needs; everything is present in the way it should be. There is a physical, therefore automatic, connection to the mother's body, which provides security and saturation: hunger, thirst, and sleepiness are naturally sated without effort or having to ask. Life, within the boundaries of the placenta (which are, though, unknown to the baby), is protected and free, within an environment that is perfectly fitting, warm, and welcoming.

Not even a disabled child registers any discomfort in the womb, because there is nothing in the environment that exceeds his capabilities. If we want to look for evidence of omnipotence in human life (not of real omnipotence, of course, but of a perceived omnipotence), we can definitely find it in the infant's experience within the womb. Only birth will precipitate the baby into the world of limits, the entering of which, however, the baby is, and should be, totally oblivious of at the time. I often think that without the experience of life within the womb, and of the total, blissful saturation that marks it, we could not explain the human quest for happiness. We pursue it because we have felt it. We could not imagine it, had we not somehow experienced it.

For a long time, it has been thought that a baby in the womb is too immature, both physically and emotionally, to register anything. Such was the certainty that, until recently, having to carry out painful manoeuvres on premature newborns with the intent of keeping them alive, doctors operated without anaesthesia in the belief that the fibres which transmit pain had not been activated yet. Still, many such babies inexplicably died, and only later did physicians realise that they suffered heart attacks because of the pain. They also discovered that the best anaesthetic was, in fact, the presence of the mother or a substitute who knew how to hold and contain the baby: whispering soothing words into the baby's ear, slipping something sweet into the baby's mouth. This, in other words, amounts to re-creating a perceptual matrix that resembled the recent experience of the womb, saturating the infant's senses exactly as used to happen within the maternal affective container of the womb. The pain would then not be registered, as the tender holding provided sensory saturation that filled up the baby's perceptual capabilities. This observation substantiates the hypothesis that the baby experiences a specific state of complete well-being pre-birth, and that soothing after birth is much more effective if we try and reproduce a similar template of sensory stimulation (Bellieni, 2004).

Having said this, it is the amount of data that can be processed, rather than the sensitivity to perceptual data, which is limited in a newborn. On the contrary, nowadays, thanks to research with ultrasound technology, we are aware that the baby's capacities for perception and orientation are already extremely precocious within the womb. This could already be surmised by close observation of the newborn and an appraisal of his extraordinary competence in living.

The senses of touch, taste, smell, hearing, and vision slowly develop in this order, starting from the first weeks of gestation, confirming and supporting the precocity of proprioceptive sensations (Nathanielsz, 1992; Relier, 1993; Righetti & Sette, 2000; Verny et al., 1981).

However, it is worth bearing in mind that this should not be mistaken as an anticipation of the child's capacity for relatedness, that is, the ability to relate with an other-from-self. This only develops gradually after birth and will be a conquest, the fruit of a patient and demanding process in the relationship between child and carer. For the baby, mother is initially only an environment, a "state", a pleasurable being inside, an experience of physical and emotional well-being. This state of things will continue for a few months following childbirth. The baby will be naturally inclined to seek the same state of pleasure experienced while in the womb, which is the only experience he knows and the point from which, through progressive experiential expansion, his capacity for contact with the world of life will gradually be born.

What the father feels

During pregnancy, the father figure is not yet directly physically involved with the child. Still, father and child communicate indirectly by way of the physical and emotional filter of the mother figure.

The father has, in fact, a fundamental role in supporting the maternal "regression". He acts as a necessary point of reference, a custodian of rationality and experience, a support which prevents the unit constituted by mother and baby from "falling over" as a consequence of the loss of its centre of gravity. As we have seen, during gestation the mother is called upon to gradually fall into the baby's orbit: physically, as her belly swells, but emotionally, too. The same will be the case for several months following birth. The paternal presence will, instead, emerge from the symbiotic mother–child perception as a third party in his own right only gradually. The father will, in fact, have the fundamental role of being the emotional referent who tenderly supports and encourages the separation from mother and who will later guide the child's emotional world toward new terrains and goals, outside the maternal constellation.

In the course of human evolution, we can see the importance of the male figure and of his role growing proportionally to the greater degree of complexity afforded to individual development through the ages.

In our evolution, we can first note how the frequency of a woman's ovulation and human mating habits changed, so that, at a certain point, making love for humans became no longer essentially directed at procreation. Animals do not make love; they mate, guided by instincts, and for them there is no chance of wilfulness, choice, and, therefore, no project. Instead, in humans, we find that sexuality is—or should be—the supreme expression of the attainment of emotional maturity. A level of emotional development, that is, which is gained through the slow transformation of the individual's attachment needs from the world of childhood dependence to one of adult reciprocity.

Sexuality, therefore, becomes not only aimed at procreation, but an important means of emotional encounter in adult romantic attachment: a way to get to know each other, to choose and love each other, to discover a sense of unison and meeting. This all stands apart from reproductive goals, up until that certain moment when the couple finds itself harbouring a new wish: the desire that this profound and passionate union might produce something that will survive it and bring forth the priceless legacy of a felicitous encounter.

This means that, at the human evolutionary level, mating for procreation—no longer just an instinctual mechanism for the survival of the species—implies the awareness and ability to make a choice supported by a desire. Moreover, a thorough reading of Darwin's evolutionary theory itself makes this "ethical" leap a natural one. It can, in fact, be seen as an outcome of the process of becoming and transformation which permeates reality; a reality that appears moved forward by an evolutionary process whereby biology invariably develops towards ever-increasing levels of complexity and efficacy (Bertirotti, 2008, 2009; de Waal, 1996; Tinbergen, 1951). Procreation, therefore, implies our conscious adhesion to a project which is natural, yet requires, at the human level of complexity, our considered and wilful participation. Consciousness and free will, principal human attributes, must be accompanied, when deciding to try for a baby, by the couple's awareness and recognition that both motherhood and fatherhood entail an involvement which is longer and greater than in any other species. The educational commitment for a human child's evolutionary success—for him to be able to learn to adequately look after himself and to know how to be a happy and responsible adult— is very extended, requires great effort, extreme availability, and conspicuous self-sacrifice, equal to, or greater than, any other endeavour in life. This applies to father and mother alike.

The involvement of the man, his physical and emotional presence and availability for support, his gratefulness to the woman for choosing him to be the father of her child, his ability to put up with and love the physical and emotional changes his partner goes through—including her symbiotic withdrawal for the child's protection; and, ultimately, his acceptance of the fact that he is not the protagonist but a knowing and sharing accomplice, are all determining elements for a happy, successful pregnancy.

The emotional experience of childbirth: mother, father, and child

Just as a woman is passive during pregnancy (in the sense that the care and protection of the baby are automatic, without the need for her direct input), by the same token it is not the mother who decides the time of childbirth. This occurs without the mother's control, and its timing remains something located in the intimate and secret communication between the child and mother's body-selves, the outcome of the physical and emotional process which naturally edges the unit towards the relinquishing of uterine symbiosis in favour of a new form of relatedness for which the baby is now ready.

Generally, the signals in obstetrics most commonly considered as a warning that delivery is drawing near are the loss of the mucus plug—which, until this moment, has sealed the neck of the uterus, isolating it from the outside world—and the flattening and shortening of the cervix, measured by hand through simple vaginal exploration. More eloquent still is the mother's feeling of exhaustion, of having had enough, which emotionally prepares even the most reluctant of mothers to let go of their baby and get ready to meet and welcome him in another way. It is easy enough to notice when a woman enters this state by the look on her face: an unmistakable look of tiredness and exhaustion that, in ancient times, the village elders knew how to recognise and interpret as an infallible prophecy, just as they knew how to predict the phases of the moon.

This emotional sensation of tiredness and saturation is very important because it accompanies and facilitates separation, indeed making it desirable. Its arousal makes childbirth a process marked by a mix of emotions, a coalescing of feelings of desire and of loss. This powerful mix will later accompany every successive step of separation and increased individual autonomy gained within the relationship between mother and child as he grows up.

If the mother, when close to delivery, feels that she has had enough, so, too, must the baby feel increasingly cramped in the uterus, as his growth has gradually turned it into too tight a space to hold him comfortably. He will be the one, in fact, who, spurred by an unease which mirrors the mother's exhaustion, gives the first overt signals of his desire to get out. Apparently, it is the baby that, when his organism is ready, stimulates the complex neurophysiological dialogue with the mother's body which starts the paced contractions of labour (Odent, 1988). The baby, seeking a more welcoming place for his head in order to feel more comfortable, extends his short legs and places his feet against the base of the uterus: a process I like to think of, more prosaically, as a "walking" on the surface of the womb in search of a better position. This very motion creates a stimulus which, first lightly then gradually more cadenced, ends up impressing a sort of rhythmic dance on the uterine wall, with an increasingly rapid alternation of tension and relaxation. It is as if the walls of the womb began contracting following the rhythm impressed by the child and then continued of their own accord in a series of contractions and relaxations aimed at helping the baby to reach the exit. I like to think of childbirth as a precise dance, a series of alternate moments of embrace and of relinquishment, a rupture-and-repair process, the repetition of a separation tried out and then undone over and over again until only at last can it be achieved. It is an extraordinary process, this secret communication between mother and child, this synchronicity of feeling and moving gradually accompanying the dyad towards the adventure of change.

The maternal musculature involved in the contractions is an involuntary one. This means the woman cannot intervene directly on the labour process; she can only listen to it, "ride it", and let it work, trusting the natural design which through this rhythmic pressure gently pushes the baby towards the exit. The woman in labour has to follow the contraction, bear it, and then let herself surrender to, and take advantage of the restorative and painless pause that occurs at every contraction's end. A woman who is trusting and relaxed will be able to sleep and even dream during these pauses, as reported to me by a woman in childbirth. Labour is underscored by a complex and precise mechanism. The process of contractions and relaxation is underlain by the alternate release of oxytocin and endorphins, creating an extraordinary balance between exertion and relaxation, pain and blissful surrender, where the apex, the acute phase of one triggers the occurrence of the other. Alternating increasingly quickly, these phases are controlled by the brain, yet ruled by the emotions (Schmid, 2011).

Certainly, the contractions of the womb's walls are painful. The reason is simply mechanical. This essentially hollow container must be emptied of its contents and it does this by stiffening its walls, which, in turn, stretches the neck of the uterus. Initially, between every contraction, nature provides long breaks, which only very gradually shorten over time. The pauses will become longer again—to counterbalance the greater intensity of the contractions—in the final phase of expulsion.

It is much easier to let oneself take the opportunity of these moments to let go and catch some rest—letting nature run its course without resistance—if one is informed and trusting, and if the mood and surrounding atmosphere are peaceful. Odent underlines the fact that childbirth is an emotional event controlled by the right hemisphere of our brain, the same hemisphere that is more developed in the infant at birth and which will continue to be dominant for the first two years of his life (Odent, 1980). When the right brain is dominant in the processing of information, we register environments emotionally rather than analytically. The atmosphere in which the delivery occurs should, therefore, be an emotionally adequate place. Odent recommends quietness, the use of music, semi-darkness, and the absence of verbal stimuli liable to move the event to a level of intellectual control. Intellect and rationality, the "masculine" and technical, must be kept backstage and in waiting while nature and emotions are left to express themselves, yet the former must also be ready to come back on stage if and when circumstances really call for it.

Embodied in the care provision during labour and delivery, we should find the same balance that, as we shall see later on, will characterise the caring provision for the child, expressed in the complementarity of paternal and maternal templates. For the mother to be able to facilitate and accompany her child through the adventure of birth and, later on, provide the environment appropriate to each of the child's developmental stages (that is, for the mother to learn how to wait, be patient, encourage and support her child's efforts without unnecessary impingements), she, in turn, needs first to be contained and supported *herself* through participation and encouragement from those around her, especially during childbirth. Appropriate environments inspire and model the proper template of care, and good care facilitates good outcomes.

Because of its very nature, childbirth ought to be a choral event, the celebration of a new life that is about to face existence, and not something aseptic and solitary. Like the child, the mother also needs to be accompanied with patience, with the capacity to understand and share her suffering and participate in her joy. Even though in pregnancy and childbirth—events which are physiological—a woman cannot be considered a sick patient, it is, nevertheless, true that her fragility and sensibility increase considerably not only because of the labour pains, but throughout the pregnancy. This is because of the normative regression to her childhood emotional apperception of the world, as has been detailed in previous sections. This, in turn, calls upon whoever is caring for her to adopt the same sensibility, the same willingness to attune to, participate, and guide: in other words, to exercise a parental role. It is widely known that direct and exclusive involvement on the part of a midwife will immediately lower the probability of having to perform a caesarean section or even to make use of epidural anaesthesia. A strong, healthy affectivity should, therefore, be interwoven with midwifery skills in our delivery rooms.

*   *   *

Labour is generally a lengthy business, especially with the first child, and should not be rushed by external demands for cost efficiency. The reason for this slowness is, as is always the case in physiological processes, both physical and emotional. A child takes a long time to come out because this way the transition from the womb to the outside world is protected. Moreover, the slowness of labour is protective of the baby from a physical point of view, readying his vital organs to start functioning on their own (Rapisardi, 2005).

In healthy development, momentous transitions in life always occur very gradually. Thus, during labour, a child may take hours to cover just a few centimetres. His up-and-down motion not unlike the rhythmic movements of making love, allows him to slowly come to gradual contact with the new world to which he will have to adapt. The natural process indicates that the child should be gently pushed by the bottom towards life outside, rhythmically encouraging him onwards and then letting him return for a while, as if to enjoy a respite—the reassuring warmth and security of a known place which has become uncomfortable but has not disappeared—before he will be ready to try again and leave it of his own accord. The very same emotional back-and-forth motion will mark every subsequent stage of growth in life, or it should, because this is the very way human beings develop: by short hops, little bits of experience which coalesce, through repetition, into a sudden capability to leap forward, which in turn opens the way for the achievement of some greater form of competence (Brazelton & Greenspan, 2001). I like to think this imprinting to be the very great lesson of childbirth: the meaning of the alternation between effort and rest, and the opportunity to fully appreciate the great importance, both physically and emotionally, of the pauses between each contraction that quietly prepare and prompt the next effort.

Nature performs this operation throughout the whole of labour, leaving to the mother the ultimate achievement at the end, when the baby is about to come out. By then, in fact, the woman has had the opportunity to read her own body and, therefore, know how to repeat the lesson learnt, this time volitionally. This occurs not only in the ultimate pushes, but also later on, at an emotional level, in facilitating her child's developmental leaps.

Finally, the slowness of labour protects what would be an otherwise abrupt transition, physically and emotionally. The baby's slow transit from the womb toward a new life is in fact felt by the woman as an increasingly definite presence, a way to accompany and protect her from the feeling of an otherwise sudden loss. This is often the cause of experiencing a sense of intense let-down in so many women who have had a caesarean section. Therefore, the slowness of childbirth constitutes a precious opportunity to pass from the visceral perception of a baby's presence to the discovery of a different, active form of relatedness that will make up and comfort her for the loss of that deep, muffled, mysterious company which she has felt within herself for months.

* * *

During labour, as we have already detailed, the woman is "passive" in the sense that nature acts upon her without giving her conscious will the chance to stand in the way of the event. When the time of birth comes, for the survival and well-being of mother and baby, nature assertively says: separation is what must happen.

When it comes to the actual contractions, the only thing a woman can do is to go along with them, trustingly let them work, just as other animals do. She might feel tired, heavy, and uncomfortable, but she will collaborate willingly if she is properly informed and can emotionally participate in the necessity of the contractions' function. Which is no simple matter, because what has been united for nine months must now be separated.

Labour is a matter of facilitating a change of state, a new level of relatedness with the baby, which is certainly desirable and desired. However, as in every instance in life where giving up a known state (even if it has grown uncomfortable) becomes necessary, change is always received with ambivalence. On the one hand, it is wished for, but, on the other hand, feared for its novelty and tinged with melancholy as it marks the irrecoverable loss of something past. In the case of childbirth, this "something lost" is nothing less than the blissful feeling of being together in a unit that will never be the same again. Even though we are not able, or even wanting, to stop the fascinating adventure of life, a veil of nostalgic melancholy always accompanies the sense of the passing of time. With regard to this inescapable emotional fact, I feel we should take a leaf out the poets' book, letting their words stand not only as pretty distractions, but as models of staying with our emotions, even nostalgia, learning to savour the unavoidable loss that comes with development. Only in owning this can we feel the priceless sublimation that comes with the preciousness and irreplicable nature of each moment of our lives.

Therefore, if the physical pain of childbirth can be ascribed to the extension and compression of tissue, its psychological roots and justification are more complex. It is the pain that has to come with the giving up of a period of omnipotent possession to leave room for the baby's own encounter with life. The mother will still be there in a vitally important role, but she will no longer be omnipotent, that is, able to uniquely satiate each and every one of the baby's needs and desires.

So, the pain of childbirth has a profoundly emotional significance. It represents and accompanies a crucial passage: it is, in fact, an act of physical separation, of letting go, that makes possible and concrete the baby's process of individuation, already begun during intrauterine life thanks to his uniquely creative chromosome set.

Thus, inscribed in labour there is also the painful mark of the end of an era: the giving up of that total possession and constant presence which came to the mother as a blissful consolation for the inherent solitude of existing as individuated beings; in childbirth we find, instead, the expression of a maternal template different from the one the woman could feel and embody in gestation, but which represents its sustainable expression as time progresses: that is, in life. It is a maternal template which still contains but which cannot and should not retain. Labour pains deeply convey to the woman and imprint the profound perception that the life carried in the womb is not there for the keeping. The fusion with the maternal figure is only temporary and childbirth will sanction the baby's adventure in life through a slow but inevitable separation that will lead him from dependence to emancipation. I often think that no other sensation but pain could guarantee such heightened concern and concentration on the deeply meaningful task at hand, and on its lesson.

Through childbirth, a woman discovers she is only the place where, and the means through which, a destiny is accomplished. She is the conscious instrument of a natural causality the effects of which are meant to go beyond her own personal existence. For the mother, as for the baby, this change occurs through a process of leaving each other and then being reunited in a different and fascinating new relationship. Protecting and facilitating the quality of meeting will, from now on, be actively demanding, as it will be immersed, like everything else, in the precariousness of everyday life and in the ever-changing passing of time.

The emotional feeling of fatigue and weariness typical of the last phases of childbirth, which accompanies and renders the separation possible by making it feel actually desired, imbues childbirth with a mixture of emotions, as I have already explained: desire and loss, alternating pain and pleasure.

The same mixture of feelings, as I said before, will occur again at every stage of transition of the mother and child relationship. There again she will feel the wearying effect of the passing of time and the consummation of an era marked by a template of emotional related-ness that used to be blissful, but which can no longer be sustained in the same form. I am thinking, for example, of the transition from mother's milk to baby food, of the first days of kindergarten, then school, and so on until the driver's license, the diploma, all the way up to the child's achievement of financial and emotional independence. However fantastic, desired, encouraged, applauded, and sincerely shared by the mother these accomplishments on the child's part may be, there remains for her an unmistakable gloom, a nostalgia for what has passed and will not return. A mother, if true to her feelings, will, in fact, feel, amid the joy and pride, an acute sense of loss for a time, a phase, that has ended. This will seem, then, to have elapsed so quickly as to transform the fatigue, apprehension, involvement, commitment, and delight of the phase that needs to be relinquished into a memory that, like a fresco, cannot bring back the details of the single moments, however intense each was when experienced.

These are real, healthy feelings that accompany and surround our existence. They must be recognised, accepted, and shared because they mirror each other in the mother and child's experience. Much more than fatherhood, motherhood is made up of possession and nostalgia. These emotions are not aimed at withholding or impeding, but at understanding and accepting that the need to grow and the effort to change are always accompanied by ambivalence: desire and fear, curiosity and regret, conflicting feelings that can and must coexist as the mark of the wealth and power of our emotional lives.

After the forewarning signals announcing that the time has come—sometimes occurring over a period of days—the contractions start suddenly, no matter where you are or what you are doing; they are involuntary and unavoidable, marked by the lack of negotiability that signals a top priority: a modality which already anticipates the undeniable urgency that will characterise the infant's need for his mother in the weeks after birth.

This ungovernable immediacy, the impossibility of procrastinating or resisting the contractions, is designed to be overwhelming, conspicuously more irresistible than other fundamental physical needs such as hunger, thirst, sleep, or the need to urinate and defecate. This physical and emotional connotation is of the greatest importance, as it forewarns the woman of the irreducibility of the baby's need for her: not just the need to be born, but also the need to be cared for, listened to, and understood, according to rhythms and modalities that will initially have the same emotional urgency the woman experiences in the contractions. Only slowly, in fact, through time, will the initial urgency of the neonate's needs be shaped and transformed into the capacity to wait and, eventually, for intersubjective exchange.

Many intensely personal factors come into play in the capacity of a woman to withstand physical pain: her temperament, history, awareness, trust in herself and life, the emotional quality of her family heritage, and, importantly, also the modality the care provision takes during labour. The threshold of pain is not the same for everybody and can change depending on the circumstances.

Certainly, in labour it is useless and detrimental to try to fight the pain as if it were an enemy. It is more useful to see it as a fellow traveller who must be understood and allowed to act, as midwifery wisdom knows so well, so that it can perform its guiding role in the pace and positions of labour, facilitating the baby's descent towards birth.

Moreover, not only during pregnancy but above all during childbirth and the post-partum period, hormonally and emotionally driven regression can significantly bear upon the mother's availability to make use of her acquired skills. Only being able to rely on a good internalised sense of self-esteem can then make one able to cope with adversities and overcome them.

At the end of labour, which can last several hours, when the neck of the uterus has given in to the rhythmic impulses aimed at opening it up and it is completely dilated and fully effaced (even the womb needs to be coaxed into giving up its precious fruit) and when the baby's tiny head can be glimpsed at the end of the vaginal passage, *only then* can the mother act. The woman is encouraged here to add her own volitional abdominal muscle strength to the natural wave that guides the baby. Finally, urged on by the expulsive impulses of her womb, she can act and contribute to the effort of pushing her baby out, with the liberating feeling that, after so many hours, the moment of separation has arrived.

Let us take a moment to think about this. Seemingly paradoxically, the first voluntary action a mother can perform toward her child is one of expulsion. In this way, in a powerful but challenging act of separation, a process that symbolically began with nine long months of containment comes full circle. We can now fully take in how, both physically and emotionally, the cycle of pregnancy can be seen to describe and outline the full meaning of "the maternal". A mother is someone who protectively contains, but also inexorably pushes towards life. Using her own "masculinity" (the masculine aspect of herself that she carries in her emotional, neurological, and hormonal makeup) in an act of generous liberation and bequest, she has to forsake a total, perennial possession of her creature. As with the hormones, the "masculine" balances out and creates a boundary to the "feminine". Without this boundary, there would be no survival. "Masculine" and "feminine" templates are integrated to guarantee and protect life. They are the biological and affective foundations of human existence. Only through knowledge of, and respect for, these two innate complementary templates—each with its specific agenda, each the depositary of a specific set of needs and a specific repertoire of emotional patterns, but both equally necessary for survival—can man build a culture and a society able to nurture the world and act upon it without destroying.

Nature has hormonally endowed and experientially prepared the woman during pregnancy to be the one who knows how to contain and let go, taking comfort and contentment in the new phase of her relationship with her baby that starts after childbirth; she will not be alone in managing this period, though her role in the first stages is, again, unique. The baby's horizon will slowly expand to include the father and then the rest of the family and the surrounding environment, but only over time.

During the phase of expulsion, it is the mother who encourages the baby to leave his den. She does this by actively pushing, not just once, but time and again. This repetition seems to answer the need to settle this fundamental, unnegotiable, embodied imprinting properly in the mother's mind before she can move on. Her body has already taught her, through the experience of gestation, that the baby must be welcomed, protected, and surrounded by care because this is what gives him security; however, labour tells her that her baby's destiny is to detach, get out, and gradually move from dependence to emancipation. This separation, however painful, must take place in a prescribed manner. As during labour, the child must be gently nudged toward life, encouraged with a pushing out which is both supportive and liberating. The expulsive process must then again proceed by means of a slow, rhythmic pace, allowing the child at each thrust to retreat, refuel by feeling the comfort of a known environment again, and recover enough strength to stick his head out once more, this time further.

It could be argued that only after having impressed this lesson in the embodied rhythm of labour, nature can pass the baton to the mother's conscious self in the final thrusts, having shown her the way to progress in the new relationship with her child: at first complete adherence, then a slow, gradual separation.

* * *

Childbirth, the transition from symbiosis to relatedness, has both mother and child as its main performers. But they are not the only ones. If the child's environment is his mother, the mother's environment is her partner, her attachments, and the social and cultural environment of the community where she lives. Childbirth is a private event, but also a collective, social, family event. Accordingly, it is inevitable that the way society sees, interprets, and supports maternity and attachment will have a strong influence on the woman's experience.

But let us begin with the most proximal container, considering first of all that the new relationship between mother and child originates in another relationship. Birth is not a private matter between mother and child because nature has not planned for parthenogenesis. From the perspective of our evolutionary design—what nature prepared us for—the baby would not exist and the woman would not be able to be a mother had it not been for an emotional and sexual relationship. Therefore, there is always a "masculine" element, either present or implied, that participates, contains, and gives meaning.

In physiology, the support and complicity on the part of the partner in this procreative project plays a fundamental role in fostering a positive outcome. As has already been said, the symbiotic relationship between mother and child needs a watchful presence, which facilitates the covert and delicate encounter between mother and foetus as felt presence during gestation through his understanding and protective presence, thereby granting his woman the freedom to securely withdraw into herself. The father, at this stage, is asked to allow and tolerate the mother's concentration on her own internal process and her dreamy regression, even though this can deprive him of the exclusive and dedicated attention he has long enjoyed from his partner. Therefore, the father's task is to understand and accept the fact that the same passionate, instinctive drive that has supported and fed the couple's kinship and closeness beforehand has now to be devoted to supporting his child.

At childbirth, the woman is concentrated and captivated by the physicality of the event: all her companion can do is to be with her, ecstatically admiring what is happening partially thanks to him and for him, patiently reserving the pleasure of a more active complicity for the next phase. I believe the father's presence in the delivery room should be strongly recommended, not as a fad, but in order to be part of, officiate at, and celebrate the powerful symbolic act that is taking place under the direction of nature.

I would like the father to be next to the mother so that he could be the one to receive the baby she is pushing, with difficulty, towards life. His should be the arms that hold the baby who suddenly feels lost and uncontained, so that, symbolically and physically, the child can relinquish the security of his mother's womb under the protection of his father's presence and experience, and dare to walk into the world.

This would stand as an embodied representation of the process of transition that will later take place from the single maternal orbit to one expanded by the father's presence. It would involve the father in a way that would allow him to experience directly the emotional investment bestowed upon him by his child's birth.

This is the symbolic aspect. But, of course, many factors could stand in the way of this image being concretised and perhaps it will be not be possible for every father to actually experience and represent this symbolism in the delivery room (and he is no worse a father for this), but I believe everyone should have the opportunity and the privilege to have explained, and understand, the preciousness of his role to come.

We know little about what the baby feels during childbirth, though everything seems to be designed for his protection. Slowness and gradualness conspire to facilitate his passage and make his entrance into the world as soft as possible. There is only one moment when the baby signals that he is upset about what is happening to him. This is when, with the mother's final push, he pops out and "falls", finding himself in the void, and, with arms akimbo, the infant signals his new perception of a lack of containment. In a physiological delivery, this is the only moment when, as the baby is gently pushed outside, he appears to sense a moment of panic, but all it takes for him to immediately calm down is to feel wrapped up, hugged, and held tight again in a new containment.

The important metaphor contained in the baby's fright and his prompt soothing gives us a sense of how upsetting it can be to leave the womb and enter the complicated world of life, unless some trustworthy person is there to see us through. This specific moment of childbirth—when the baby comes out and calms down in a new welcoming embrace by the world—is so emotionally intense because it proves one can relinquish the false omnipotence of the womb and enter reality, with all its limitations and difficulties, *without* excessive pain or fear *as long as* there is someone there willing to share the way with you and not leave you alone. Hugging, cuddling, being together is a great recipe for comforting the sick, sad, or desperate, no matter what their age. Sharing is the magic means of overcoming any sort of adversity, severe as it might be. We must bear this in mind when the baby cries over some new bother. Affectionate hugging is soothing because it suggests a presence, a sense of sharing and of empathic participation.

Even for the woman, childbirth is, and remains, a happy event, not just one of pain. At the end of a long labour, the actual expulsion is accompanied by a crescendo of emotions. After all the effort of getting the baby's head through the exit—the hardest part to get through, as, however unset the bones may still be, nevertheless there is little room for compression of an infant's skull—the mother, in an intense final effort, encourages the rest of the little body out. If a woman is conscious and aware, as the baby slips out, she will experience a sublime, orgasmic feeling of physical pleasure in the sensitive parts of her genitals; a sense of emotional fullness, of pride and tenderness; an unforgettable jubilation and fullness of the senses and of the heart, envied by those who can only guess what it's like; a sensation that will indissolubly bond the mother to the birth of *that* child, impressing an inextinguishable seal that will stand for the rest of their lives. For those who have more than one child, there is no confusion between one birth and another. Every baby is born his or her own way; every emotion felt in childbirth is unrepeatable, and jealously stored in memory.

Pain and pleasure, therefore, chase and balance each other out. To consider childbirth only as a brutally painful experience is a clear sign of our society's inability to grasp the depth and emotional complexity of this extraordinary event.

Another important thing to consider as a factor hindering or facilitating a delivery is the fact that the mother can trustingly let her baby out only if she feels that she is putting him in a safe place. And, as in the moment of expulsion she cannot entirely provide for the baby by herself, her partner is, ideally, the person she will be able to trust to share this new responsibility with. The father's role at that moment will become actualised for the first time: that is, to be there to widen the protective circle with his own presence, in due course encouraging the little one to leave his mother, trust himself, and feel secure to lean out towards the real world because his father is there waiting for him, leading him by the hand and showing him the way.

Note how there is an exchange of roles at childbirth. The woman, aligned with her "masculinity", is intent on expelling, pushing out, and distancing herself from her baby; the man is busy receiving, replacing the mother with his own "femininity" to protect and escort the child. All this has a counterpart in masculine or feminine hormonal peaks that can be measured.

So, it is at the moment of childbirth that we have the first enactment—embodied in both the symbolic and factual levels—of the complementarity and integration of masculine and feminine templates necessary to caregiving. Even in his life after childbirth, the baby will be pushed out from the maternal containment towards conquering greater self-reliance and autonomy with an alternating movement—as in childbirth—between exploration of the unknown and return to the known. This dynamic will be based on, and made secure by, both the paternal and maternal presence.

In order to better represent the complementary relationship between feminine and masculine, I often use the graphic image used in set theory to describe two intersecting sets (Figure 2.1).

Male and female overlap in an area made up of the male element in a woman and the female element in a man. The child develops here in this area. If, at the beginning of life, in pre-birth and post-partum, the maternal world prevails as an adequate, sufficient container that is welcoming and protective, *then* as the baby grows older he will be able to move forward securely into an area where the paternal sphere integrates the maternal. The paternal world will operate as a widening and integration of the maternal constellation, promoting a confident separation, which will lead the child onwards towards a slow, gradual acquisition of autonomy.

A painting comes to mind, certainly more evocative than the intersecting sets of Figure 2.1: Giorgione's *The Tempest* (Fornari, 1981) (Figure 2.2). This splendid and intriguing picture has long kept scholars and critics engaged in a quest to decipher its alleged occult

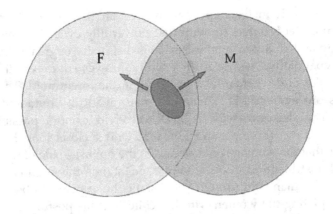

Figure 2.1. The feminine–masculine complementarity.

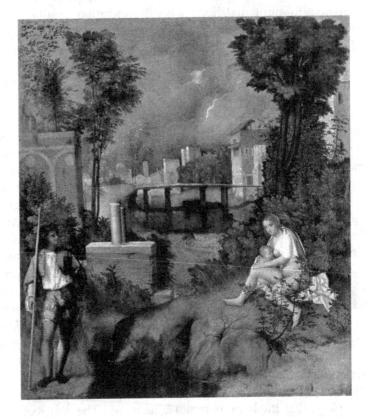

Figure 2.2. *The Tempest,* by Giorgione.

symbolisms. It instead appears to me that this piece of artwork uncomplicatedly refers to, with that powerfully evocative emotional strength and ability to synthesise that is distinctive of great artists, the archetypal natural family. At first sight, our eyes are captured by the image of a nude woman and her child in the foreground. The dyad stands out against a backdrop of a naturalistically rendered land-scape. This strikes us with its bleak, yet vivid, colours, possibly still wet after a recent tempest (childbirth?). Only a closer look, however, reveals that the woman is not alone. On the opposite side of the paint-ing, almost blended into the landscape, stands the slightly shaded figure of a man. Withdrawn yet ecstatic, he appears to be humbly contemplating the woman with her child. But his posture and cloth-ing, half peasant attire and half soldier's uniform, both indicate he is ready to move, to intervene should anything unexpected happen. I have always thought that here, with the intuition, synthesis, and eloquence of a truly great artist, Giorgione represented and antici-pated an entire psychoanalytical treatise.

Post-partum: a renewed bonding

Immediately after childbirth, the newborn, lying on his mother's belly, slowly but relentlessly crawls up toward the nipple. Nowadays, when women from different countries and cultures have children in our hospitals, we know that babies can recognise their own mothers from the taste of their colostrum and then their milk. Scents connected to the mother's unique smell and her diet have, in fact, already left traces in the taste of the amniotic liquid.

This instinctive search that pushes the baby up towards the nipple is supported by important and complex neurobiological reactions. It would seem the incentive to reach the nipple is tied to a build-up of catecholamine during childbirth that spurs the baby to seek comfort from the adrenalin-induced stress by sucking from the mother's breast, subsequently releasing endorphins for both the mother and child (Volta, 2006). Notice how everything we do for the survival of our species is accompanied by pleasure.

The most common belief regarding this apparent urgency to grasp the nipple is that the baby is hungry; he is not. The real reason the baby seeks to reunite with his mother lies in the need to regain and rekindle the symbiosis. Once the baby has terminated the period of passive connection, that is, the period of life inside the womb, a new stage of active symbiosis begins. During this phase, mother and child must commit actively, though still instinctively, to recreate that unity which, in childbirth, was broken only physically, whereas emotionally the dyad is still very much symbiotically connected.

As I have said, childbirth is not a beginning, but just a moment of transition: a passage from a passive bond, requiring no effort—on the part of either the baby or the mother—to an active bond, but still a symbiotic one. Indeed, after childbirth, it is the baby, driven by his own innate preparedness for symbiosis, who actively searches to re-establish connection to his mother's body through sucking from her breast, an innate instinct which he has already rehearsed in the womb, sucking his thumb or hand or even toe through sixteen long weeks. In the mother's complementary hard-wired preparedness, this action stimulates and increases the production of colostrum, triggered even before childbirth, and then milk. Since she has been recognised and chosen by the taste of her milk, smell of her body, and sound of her voice (which the baby has perfectly registered through her womb), it will then be the mother's task, however, to actively and intentionally foster this activity, already familiar to the baby. This comes fairly naturally, but *only* if the mother can rely on an internalised confidence in her ability to learn by practice, on the one hand, and to nourish, on the other.

There is no greater despot than a newborn. Convinced he is still inside the womb—since he has no other experience—he expects everything to work as before, easy and enjoyable. Therefore, he indignantly protests about anything he finds in any way unpleasant, any disturbance to the state of bliss to which he is accustomed. The world into which the baby is born is so utterly new to him, and governed by such different rules, that only very gradually can he grow to understand and become adapted to it.

The natural design does not, in fact, plan for a sudden, quick loss of this pre-life state of grace, destined to act as the asymptotic horizon of happiness, but, rather, for its initial substitution by a world of physical and emotional care capable of holding him. This will stimulate and facilitate the child's development to gradually open the way for his active and more and more direct contact with reality. Only if this process takes place gradually and lovingly will the child-become-adult truly be able to understand, not only cognitively but emotionally, the world, and face it without the distorting shadow of a premature, traumatic loss of basic trust in that same world.

In a metaphor similar to the English "born with a silver spoon in one's mouth", Italians say that a lucky baby is born with a shirt. I find this popular expression evocative, as, in a sense, the infant is wrapped in a sort of protective envelope. First, the immaturity of his senses protects him from what would otherwise be an overwhelming cacophony of stimuli thanks to a high threshold of perception; second, with her loving care, his mother can easily saturate the processing capacities of his young brain with pleasurable sensations, providing him with the emotional illusion of still being inside the womb. As has been said, from the perspective of the emotional connection between mother and baby, childbirth is not the final word, but, rather, just a moment of transition. For the infant, being born is only the prelude within the gradual process of gaining a sense that his mother and he are two separate selves and not one: everything has yet to be done. Emerging from symbiosis, or "hatching", actually occurs only a relatively long time after birth, and the active function of parents—first the mother, then both—will be vital for the child's individuality as a separate subject to have the chance to come into being at all.

It will take a long, patiently borne time, as in childbirth, for the newborn baby to begin to comprehend the change that has taken place and learn to trust the new environment in which he finds himself. The mother figure is, again, crucial for the baby to complete this transition in a non-traumatic way, that is, in a way that is attuned and adapted to his (im)maturity. Initially, she has to create around the baby an emotional environment able to convey what Winnicott calls the "initial illusion" (Winnicott, 1958) of still being in the womb. Enveloped by her care and following a timing attuned to the thresholds set by his necessarily slow neurobiological development, the mother should then let her baby gradually emerge from his sensory and emotional "protective wrap" towards the unfiltered perception of his new reality.

From the hormonal point of view, it is prolactin that acts on the mother in the very first weeks to make her inclined and able to provide the absolute, contingent availability needed then by the child.

It now becomes apparent why nature has designed delivery to be just the way it is: its lengthiness, gradualness, and the effort and patience involved, fully acquire their sense as an embodied template of care, outlining a model of how biological development unwinds which must be respected and actively fostered after birth. The same forward-and-backward dynamics will also characterise the baby's developmental process and the same template of care expressed in childbirth will have to inform the parents' provision.

The imprinting of childbirth becomes a particularly crucial guideline as it helps the mother perform her new active task of moving the child from renewed symbiosis to physical and emotional separation, gently *pushing* him towards the slow, gradual building of his identity. She will be the one to encourage her child towards separation through the little conquests he achieves on a daily basis, reassured by the mother figure through change that would otherwise be frightening, and nourished by the milk which fuels his body's growth.

Contrary to what we culturally assumed for a long time, the more mother and child benefit from their renewed emotional symbiosis, the easier it will be to separate later on. This is because the child has a natural tendency to take in and master reality, as well as explore it, as time passes and his physical and emotional development allows it. Indeed, some athletic ability will eventually be useful if you want to keep up with him.

This is one of the reasons nature has set a fertility threshold and women can no longer have babies after a certain age. But it is fundamental that, alongside his vitality, there should also be respect for the child's extreme fragility, his absolute need to feel seen, loved, and wanted by caring parents. If this is already true in the animal world, though in a more instinctive and unaware way, certainly the perception of being lovingly cared for acquires an indisputable importance for human beings. This is because, in our species, it is the bond, the attachment, which triggers in the infant a sense of security as opposed to experiencing annihilating terror. This is not just in infancy: this need for the love of the other (in more complex forms than symbiosis, as we shall see) to feel secure will be part of us for all our lives. Attachment and its inherent sense of dependable security must, therefore, be fostered immediately after birth, so that a solid base for future growth and separation is established.

Few of us live in close contact with animals these days, other than the occasional pets, and these are seldom allowed to reproduce. So it is that the birth of a litter of cats or dogs is an increasingly rare event in a private home. This is a shame, as it would offer an extraordinarily effective opportunity to observe all the processes we have so far described, albeit in a condensed form: the continuing presence of symbiosis after birth, the mother's watchful protection, her complete initial dedication to the care of her offspring; then how, only little by little, she offers her puppies increasingly larger areas of experience, up until their progressive detachment, when each of the newborns has finally grown into full competence.

Labour and delivery are, therefore, not isolated events, carrying no particular meaning, which could then be manipulated at will without consequences. Childbirth is a bridge connecting two parts of a single, carefully designed, natural process that begins in the womb, where the baby begins to perceive life; until then, his care is ensured passively, through the predisposition of an environment perfectly adapted to his needs. The parents' behaviour is, or should be, the direct heir of this template of care, already begun by nature in the uterus and then in an embodied, emotional enactment in childbirth: a model which must be imitated and followed if we are to foster the full, harmonious development of a child.

A patient, considerate response

The baby reaches for the breast to restore the physical bond with his mother, which was suspended with the cutting of the umbilical cord. More than by the need to alleviate hunger, a child is bonded to his mother by an emotional need for security. Nature uses the breast, where emotional urgency is fulfilled, for passing the milk, not the other way round. The search for a physical meeting, as will be the case later, in sexuality, becomes the way of expressing attachment, the emotional bond. Milk will, therefore, become, together with the satisfaction of the senses, the mark and tangible sign of maternal care. It will be again a physical state of fulfilment signalling to the child that he is in the right place, through experiencing the continuance of that already-known quality of care he has felt in the womb, which releases a sense of pleasure and reassurance. Food, thus, acquires the emotional significance of an intermediary for motherly love, something preserved at times even into adulthood as a symptom, a recognisable sign of a longing to quench an early unfulfilment or, on the contrary, to reject an overwhelming excess of maternal concern.

In the early days marked by this passionate embrace that recreates a unity broken only physically at birth, it is senseless to think of a precise schedule for hunger and sleep. As her body accommodated pregnancy to make space for the foetus, the woman must adapt to her baby's requirements, attuning to, and standing by, his rhythms and needs, at least in the beginning. Naturally, no mother can be as perfect as her womb in responding to the initial need for bonding. However, the baby's communication skills right after birth, as archaic as they may be, in combination with a serene maternal attitude of willingness to try, can work wonders in recreating this fundamental illusion of continuance.

During his first days, the little one clings to the breast, letting go to fall asleep only when exhausted. It is a considerable effort for him to manage to suck milk through the thin milk ducts. When he reawakens, he inevitably looks for his mother again, since she is the only recognisable point of reference capable of re-evoking and rekindling the only memory he possesses: the womb. I always advise mothers to be attuned and contingently available, to promptly answer the baby's cries and avoid imposing a too sudden—and, therefore, violent—separation on the baby for fear of "spoiling" him.

I remember I once heard a newborn's spasmodic crying in the maternity ward where I worked. I could not resist and I went to see what was happening. On identifying the room, I found myself facing a woman lying half-dressed on her bed. She was observing her baby as he lay flat on his back, crying desperately, all blue in the face with the effort. The baby was regurgitating a lot of milk from both mouth and nose, so I felt I should suggest to her that perhaps her baby needed help. She looked at me covertly and, with a conniving glance, she whispered as if not to be overheard by the baby, "He's a sly one!" "What do you mean, sly?!" I asked. "When was he born?" "The day before yesterday." "How can a two-day-old baby be sly? Maybe he needs something," I suggested. And the woman, still under her breath, said, "He wants his mummy." I insisted, "What else should he want, do you think?" I picked up the baby and leaned him against my shoulder so that he could finally burp, thinking to myself what a rough time this poor thing was going to have, trying to be understood.

Concerns about "spoiling" are widespread and readily held by mothers, fathers, grandmothers, and neighbours alike; this would be a healthy concern if applied to the truly spoiled children, the older ones, whose parents are incapable of saying "no" and who are inappropriately left to do anything they want without boundaries. But a newborn baby is a different matter; answering his needs is an obligation, taking care of him is the only possible contingency available for him, after having conceived him without his actual knowledge. Commitment to a child's care must be taken into account together with the decision to procreate.

At least three months will pass before a child can understand that he is separated and become able to trust the physical separation as a still secure emotional place.

A book was published about ten years ago that was, and still is, very popular among new parents. This book compares a child to a household appliance and prompted me to start writing down these thoughts of mine, as I believe mothers dream of electric babies as much as the android of Dick's prophetic dystopia dreamt of electric sheeps. They wished for real ones. Nevertheless, in this book the author claimed that, following his "operating manual", it would be possible for parents to teach a baby how to sleep, as if the baby did not already have the skills to do that, had not already slept during the nine months of pregnancy, and had not put himself to sleep of his own accord since the moment he was born! Indeed, newborns sleep most of the time, just like in the womb. The book, however, suggests a method that consists in guiltlessly letting the baby cry and resisting the temptation of answering his calls. The same book claims that the child, from day one, must be put to sleep at 8.30 p.m. (Estivill & Anderson, 2008).[1] Nothing could be further from the truth about a baby, as becomes apparent if one just has the patience to hear, observe, and understand an infant. (For an opposing view to that of Estivill and Anderson (2008), see Honegger Fresco (2006).)

I recommend that mothers initially give their baby the breast on request, though this does not mean responding to every single one of the child's cries by feeding him. If the discomfort triggering the protest is not hunger, an infant can easily be reassured simply by holding him. The light bouncing and rocking in his mother's arms will evoke the similar motion in the womb when his mum was walking, bringing him back to something known and reassuring.

Then there is the voice. It has been proved beyond doubt that a child already knows his mother's voice from his experience in the womb, though slightly muffled as he was hearing it from the inside. It seems he also hears the father's voice through the walls of the womb in the third trimester of pregnancy. Few women are aware of the importance of the use of their voice and its quality: tone, pitch, and prosody.

In the hospital I would often hear babies crying so obstinately I felt compelled to intervene. I would then sometimes find myself in a room where a mother would be caught up in her baby's first change of diaper. The baby would be lying on the bed or changing board, half-naked and howling. The mother, completely indifferent to the baby's cries or distraught but looking lost, would appear to be concerned about the practicalities of the manoeuvre, such as which side of the diaper went where. It was usually enough for me to enter the room and ask, in an *attuned* (soft, affectionate, sing-along) tone of voice: "What's so terribly wrong for this little one to be crying like that?" and the baby would immediately stop howling, as if transfixed, captured, and start turning his head toward the voice. Without understanding a word that was spoken, the baby hears the voice, the soft tone, and immediately calms down.

It becomes easy to attune to, understand, and soothe a baby if we put ourselves in his shoes: being divested of his nappy must be an uncomfortable and disorientating experience, especially if the nappy was full of warm urine. Losing suddenly the warm containment of the nappy, the baby finds himself uncovered and "alone" with his body exposed. All it takes is to talk to him and replace the reassuring wrapping with an equally reassuring vocal "envelope" which makes him feel contained. Instead, a high, shrieking tone would certainly frighten him. There was a time when babies were wrapped up like mummies. Back in the day, it might have been more to keep them quiet, but it also made them feel secure. The practice was later dropped because it raised hygienic concerns.

If the mother's response is contingent and patient, the baby will gradually regulate his feeding times on his own, taking in greater quantities of milk and, therefore, being able to wait for longer intervals.

Gradually getting into a habit of regular feeding times is important, without forcing or imposing it too early. There are two reasons for this: physically this fosters the imprinting of a regular emptying of stomach and intestines, in line with good hygiene; emotionally, the regularity and dependability of the appointment with feeding and his mother will help the baby, unable as he is to understand the abstract notion of time—even at the age of eight children still confuse "last" with "next"—to measure the time of day through the cadenced repetition of a fulfilling emotional encounter. In other words, the rhythmical encounter with the mother's breast will offer the baby a first physical and emotional measure of time.

Among the various mammals, our species is one of those whose milk production is of relative limited amounts at a time. Again, this apparent hindrance is not accidental, but instead it supports human beings' emotional need for frequent bonding, which in turns guarantees the repeated experience of the mother figure that is required for internalisation. Indeed, only patient repetition allows for the creation of an experience that over time can become a dependable certainty, something that can be *trusted*. Every feeding time is a re-encounter. The baby wakes up disoriented, uncontained, and desperately seeks a presence; he recognises the smell, the contact, the sound of the mother's voice, and then finds the breast. Through cycles of waiting and finding, repetition and time, the child can gradually build the certainty of a presence that is external yet available, and who slowly assumes the features of the mother figure.

Therefore, the importance of breastfeeding lies not only in the better quality of maternal milk—better suited to the baby's nutritional needs and rich in antibodies to protect him from illness—but also in the emotional need for repeated experiences of separation and symbiosis. It is this reassuring pattern in fact that slowly brings the baby to recognise his mother as a separate object, yearned for, and found over and over again. It is this cycle that, in other words, from symbiosis takes the infant towards the discovery of relatedness. During and through breastfeeding, the baby gradually realises he is one of *two*. The transition from confidence through physical contact to confidence through the internalisation of his mother's presence as a separate but still dependable, secure fact, will be fundamental for the child's growth. But this will take time.

While the baby is still small, unable to understand and, therefore, cope with separation, and meals are frequent, I recommend having him sleep in a cot in the parents' room, making it easier for the mother, too, to comfortably manage night feeds while avoiding tiresome nocturnal trips to the nursery. I have been told that Sicilian peasants used to place a hammock over the parents' bed where their baby could easily be lulled to sleep if he woke up during the night. I also advise not to protect the baby's sleep from light and noise during the day, so that he can slowly learn that a good time to rest is the peace of night, thereby gradually synching his schedule to circadian rhythms. Most children are born with a "reversed" sleep pattern and swap day with night. This is due to the fact that during pregnancy their mother was mostly active during the day; as she moved about, the baby was lulled and encouraged to sleep; when the mother slept, however, the baby could wake up and move around more freely in an expanded container, made available by the mother's supine position.

During the first months of his life, a baby is in no danger of picking up bad habits. He is so small he will not be able to calculate any sort of blackmail. I prefer not to give a precise age for developmental stages. The important thing is knowing what is going to happen and why, and allowing every child to do this in his or her own time and way.

Creating a secure base and building confidence

Being able to "trust at a distance" is the most complex cognitive and emotional attainment that a baby has to reach during the first months of his life, and it is achieved by way of internalising the mother's presence. This will constitute the secure base on whose foundation it will be possible for the child to set forward with that piston-like, forwards-and-backwards movement of exploration and return I described earlier as the experiential motion with which we have all grown up and which stands at the root of development towards authentic emotional maturity. Clearly, if the experience of security remained dependent on contact with the mother's body, the baby's exploratory movements would only be able to cover very limited distance. Therefore, backed by repeated experiences of maternal availability and facilitated by the physical development of his sensory and cerebral functions, the baby must achieve a gradual separation from the physicality of his mother's care, while still feeling secure. Body-contact will be gradually substituted by a capacity to mentalize the dependability of the maternal presence, that is to *trust*. This capacity to emotionally evoke the experience of the mother's care and its soothing effect will gradually make the child feel secure even in the absence of physical contact, then slowly in the absence of her physical being.

The mental operations underlying the ability of feeling secure at a distance are extremely complex, both cognitively and emotionally, however this capacity is often taken for granted by adults. It instead requires a long period of time to be accomplished. In fact, from a certain perspective it is never fully achieved, if we consider how even we "grown-ups" still get slightly anxious when we face some of the numerous separations that we are subdued to in the course of a normal existence, let alone the traumatic ones of loss and migration.

The first step toward the achievement of this fundamental ability takes place around the third month, when we can observe the child for the first time performing *intentional* disengagement motions, which signal a first distancing from the bond with the maternal body. The timing is not random, but it coincides with a significant leap in maturation involving eyesight. This is the last of the senses to start functioning in full, in part because it is the most complex and partly since it cannot, strictly speaking, "develop" in the darkness of the mother's womb. In the first weeks, the extension of a child's focus is in fact only about thirty centimetres (twelve inches), exactly the distance between the mother's breast and her face. Generally speaking, however, though some of them are already operational at birth, *all* sensory organs still need to consolidate their perceptive abilities through experience and learning (Herbinet & Busnel, 1981; Spitz & Cobliner, 1965).

In the third month the baby is already much more involved and attentive, not exclusively focused on emptying the breast of its milk. We can observe how he gradually becomes more in control and aware of what he is doing. Even during feeds, he appears more reflective: he sucks then stops, starts sucking again, then stops again. Concentrated and absorbed, he is discovering that if he sucks, the milk comes; if he stops, no milk comes. He appears particularly pleased with this discovery. It feels as if his new-found skill makes him quite proud of his power, so to speak, or at least I would not know how else to describe the clear pleasure babies display every time they discover their own abilities.

So it happens that, at a certain moment, all of a sudden, the baby, one hand still leaning on the breast, lifts his gaze towards his mother's face with a questioning look. It feels almost as if he were asking for a sign of recognition for what is happening, the recognition of his new ability.

This happens to be one of those calls upon the carer for validation, for recognition, and for a sharing of experience, all crucial ingredients for a child's growth. Indeed, it is essential for a child to be able to pass on his emotions to the adult with whom he is relating, so that he may receive acknowledgement of his feeling in return: encouragement if this is positive, or containment if negative.

As she is breast-feeding, if attentive and involved, a mother will notice this new, significant look—simultaneously questioning and absorbed—that all of a sudden the baby is pointedly directing at her, fishing for her attention. She will then be likely to respond with a smile of satisfaction, acknowledging the competence and awareness her child has now achieved. A child at three months is already familiar with eye contact, so the baby, facing the mother's approving smile, would look even more pleased and happy at the validation received. He will subsequently dive again into the mother's soft breast, to re-emerge and re-engage his mother anew with the same proud look, to feel seen and approved of once again.

Then, at some point in this repetitive game, the baby will answer his mother's smile with a smile of his own; as he smiles he will open his mouth a little, not much but enough for him to lose grip of the nipple. He will remain that way for a moment, with milk dribbling from the corners of his mouth, "suspended" and held by the interlocking of loving glances.

For the first time, here, for a brief moment, the child willingly gives up physical contact in favour of this other embrace, this "virtual", immaterial, but intensely emotional contact, created by the meeting of the eyes.

It is the beginning of a trust that shifts from contact to connection, from symbiosis to relatedness-at-a-distance. Repeated over and over again, consistent experiences like the one described above will consolidate for the baby a deep sense of trust in the dependability of a loving maternal being-there, emotionally resonant, yet physically separate. The experience of mother, registered and mentalized as captured by the eyes and the other senses, will then be internalised as a reassuring image to accompany him in his explorations of the world and when alone.

This is the beginning of physical separation, an adventure that, thanks to the consolidation of the consistency of the mother's presence, will allow the baby to go out into life while maintaining deep inside the certainty of an attachment figure he can rely on.

All of this must still be accomplished through, and over a long span of time. This first encounter, at the mother's breast, is only the first step. Instead, it is often taken for granted that the newborn is already equipped for life and that he is only physically small, but already "sly" in his demands; or, on the contrary, he is thought of as stupid, completely unable to understand or relate with agency.

After this first intentional eye contact and this first internalisation, the baby's development really takes a leap forward. His connection with reality becomes more and more enriched and he begins to relate significantly, even to other persons he experiences, among whom, fundamentally, the father figure stands out. With the beginning of relatedness, the baby conspicuously starts to accept the father figure, to explore it with growing interest, to tolerate it as a substitute caring presence, while still maintaining his partiality for mummy.

From this moment on, the child can also start making symbolic use of objects, such as the dummy, his teddy bear, his security blanket, with beneficial effects on his growth. He will start to use them, as Winnicott says, as "transitional objects"; in other words, objects that, thanks to their sensory qualities of being soft to the touch and easy to suck, remind him of, and are capable of evoking, the motherly care he has received (Winnicott, 1971). He will take them with him when he is alone, when he is exploring new experiential spaces, or when he goes to sleep, as a talisman evoking the presence and continuous existence of his precious carer. Thanks to their power to evoke in the baby the first symbolic operation, these objects afford the child, thanks to his emotional investment in them, greater autonomy. Only once he has internalised a sufficient degree of confidence in himself and in the relationship with his parents, can the child sleep in his own room, thanks to a sense of trust which is able to "cradle" him from a distance.

Regarding this difficult conquest, namely the attainment of object-constancy, it comes as no surprise that, from this moment on until the age of one, a child's favourite game is "peek-a-boo", which involves the disappearance and reappearance of a face. This apparently mundane dynamic fills the child with such joy that he can often break out in laughter when he observes the "magical" reappearance of something that had disappeared. The baby's wonder is comparable to our own as we observe a magician's skill, though he can be much more intensely taken by his emotion. For the child, in fact, this is *actually* a miracle, but also and especially it is the cathartic repetition of a soothing cycle whereby the familiar experience of loss and anxiety triggered by absence is overcome and soothed by the reappearance of the love-object.

* * *

As I have explained, during the first three months the father figure remains a secondary figure for the baby. Even though his presence is fundamental in supporting the mother, just as his support was during her pregnancy, for the newborn dad is not, at this stage in his development, perceived as a significant presence. In this phase, an attuned father cannot do much more than replace the mother in the form of care required by a newborn, made up of support and containment, an attitude that we associate with a feminine constellation. From the onset of relatedness, however, the father, too, will be invested with a "transitional" role: an object capable of symbolically evoking the maternal presence and her care, only gradually to acquire a different, personal role: Daddy, the facilitator of detachment from mother and of exciting exploration, the confident master of "doing" and of "knowing", the god-like, superhero figure supporting the child's physical and emotional progress to independence.

Starting from the sixth month, the baby is ready to take other forms of food to supplement his diet. In the same way as with milk, at this stage a mother can no longer supply all the emotional nourishment a baby needs by herself, so that other people and other experiences must integrate her role.

It takes a long time for a baby to emerge from the safety of symbiosis because this is the length of time required to acclimatise to the operations underlying the complexity of human relational life. As in pregnancy and childbirth, parents must attune and adapt their behaviour to the child's age, respecting his timeframe and ways with participation and guidance. Without accompaniment, a child will never be able to carry out and complete the journey of development towards maturity.

It seems to me that many—too many—ignore how a child's identity is really construed. The little ones come to know and gain a sense of who they are and of the world through their relationship first with mother, then with both their parents, then with the extended family, babysitters, nursery school, and society in general. Whether we like it or not, we are all educators, and our behaviour and attitude towards the young is a great responsibility. A child has no knowledge, and has every right not to. He still has everything to learn. He experiences emotions, the first and most basic linked to his physical being, and "consigns them" to his caregivers to regulate and understand them. He has no other option but to ask for help because he is absolutely incapable of meeting his own needs or protecting himself. All his needs must be met by a caregiver. Then, when he begins to achieve a certain degree of partial competence and autonomy, he will still need an adult with whom he can share his discoveries and emotions, bestowing his "whys" upon us to have an exchange of views, to understand and learn from those who have more experience. A child requires participation and engagement.

I like to view the development of a child as the weaving of a fabric where he is the warp and we the weft. His relationship with adults is comparable to a game of catch, where his emotion or experience is "thrown" to us, and then returned to the child enriched and contained by our response. It will then be the product of this interpersonal processing of the child's experience, marked by the caregiver's response, which will be internalised by the child as a rule, a truth about the world or himself. This, in turn, will condition the child for a long time to come, perhaps even all his life, both in how to deal with his internal experience and in what that experience should comprise. This interpersonal process could also be imagined as knitting, where the yarn must pass between two needles to be woven, otherwise the structure fails and we are left with a hole, a void. Being with a small child as an emotionally available adult, the feeling is a bit like being bombarded with his sensations, emotions, experiences, and, later, thoughts (all parents are familiar with the Why? phase). He cannot help but do so because he does not yet have the means to deal with them on his own; he needs to share; he must not be ignored or, on the contrary, invaded and overwhelmed by external impingement, that is, emotional demands and needs that are not his own, but the adult's.

The more the caring is given with loving awareness of, and respect for, the child's boundaries (like the womb that *contains but does not compress* the foetus), the earlier he will be reassured that that extraordinary presence, the "goddess" who has brought him to life, the mother whom he desperately needs, the only one who can make him feel secure and whom he trusts, will still be there even if she is not present. Moreover, that the same security he knows from body-contact is felt through a different kind of connection, one that is emotional rather than physical. The more a child can be confident about the dependability of the mother's emotional availability at the beginning, the more he will be free to develop untroubled by anxiety. He will be able to enjoy the slow acquisitions which gradually emancipate him without being deprived of the basic feeling of the security of the early contact. He will then grow up not because someone needs, wants, or coerces him to, but because he can (Mahler et al., 1975; Tomasello, 2009; Winnicott, 1965b).

The slow journey towards autonomy and the father's role

I will not deal here with all the successive stages of a child's growth towards the acquisition of autonomy and emotional maturity. By this, I mean the attainment of a state of being and relating which is set by nature to be the end-point of a developmental process, a process meant to take one to a place where one achieves emotional well-being and the full creative deployment of one's own talents.

What I would instead like to focus on in this section is the fact that reaching this goal requires, alongside the child's own vital energy inscribed in his corporeity and personal talents, the concomitant presence of adequate emotional response patterns, performed by parents willing to commit to the difficult task of facilitating their child's journey towards maturity.

The stages of child development are well described in all major texts on developmental psychology or pedagogy. Instead, what I wish to really put across here is that a baby comes out of the initial state of symbiotic attachment only gradually and through a succession of crucially timed stages of emotional development, which can only occur when the previous stage's needs and goals have been fully met. It is only then that parents and children alike can suddenly find themselves confronted with a new ability, as if coming out of the blue. This is because, as we have seen, development progresses in leaps, and the leap (that is, the appearance of the new ability) takes place only when the child has already had the time and possesses the interpersonal "ingredients" required to master the abilities of the previous stage.

One example that comes easily to mind of such apparent leaps is the moment when, suddenly and unexpectedly, after much happy crawling, one day a parent finds the child, doubtful and uncertain, standing up, perhaps using the couch in the living room as leverage. Following the pattern earlier described as serving the child's need for participation and approval, the now toddler looks up into our eyes for encouragement before daring to take his first step.

Before this sudden transition to ambulation in an erect position, the baby usually crawls around for a long time, as if measuring up the surrounding environment. During the crawling phase, it is fascinating to see how, when the baby is resting and returns to a seated position, he does not normally sit with his legs apart, an instable position. Instead, he can be observed drawing a triangle with his legs by folding one of them to prop himself up and find balance. This can be seen in Figure 2.3.

We could say, then, that not only emotionally, but also physically, as any engineer knows, the magic number is three: three separate but connected elements composing a triangle, the most resilient configuration on earth. We can find the same triplicity gradually outlined with the transition from symbiosis to the discovery of the father figure.

Spitz (1965) describes the stages of child development as mediated by the time-sequenced acquisition of specific sets of experience-dependent patters of relating which in turn act as organisers of the child's internal object relations. For example, the smiling response

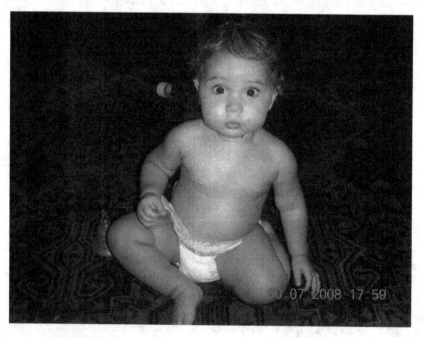

Figure 2.3.   Position a baby adopts when seated after crawling.

described earlier; the "stranger anxiety", which appears around the seventh month thanks to new perceptive abilities making it possible to discriminate between faces (searching for the mother's face and not finding it in the features of others), or the use of "no" around the eighteenth month as a way of setting a boundary between the child's will and that of others and, therefore, achieving a degree of autonomy (this one is a small taste of things to come in the distant adolescent future). All these significant leaps in development, according to Spitz and Cobliner (1965), introduce, facilitate, and consolidate a shift in the child's levels of awareness and relational capacities in the direction of higher complexity.

It is worth repeating here that children's maturation occurs in leaps, following a non-linear process whereby the exploration of reality made accessible at a certain stage by daily practice of the current capacities suddenly gives rise to a new skill, which again will be tested and rehearsed until confidence is achieved. Every cycle of exploration is followed by a return to the known, a refuelling of security, to only then being able to move further. These dynamics, as has been explained, retrace the process of childbirth (Brazelton & Sparrow, 1992, 2008).

In the physical and emotional development of a child, another crucial moment worth mentioning in some more detail is marked by the acquisition of the ability to control the sphincter and, thereby, becoming able to empty himself voluntarily. Nature places the achievement of this physical and mental skill around the third year. Before then, I warn parents, there is no use in trying to rush things for convenience's sake, as the child is simply not yet equipped to deal with this step, neither physically nor neuro-biologically. If toilet training is enforced, then it can certainly be obtained, but by conditioning, just like tricks can be learned by dogs or monkeys at the circus.

One might wonder why such a basic ability is designed to be achieved so late. The answer is: because it has great symbolic significance. Let us remember that, for the child, who cannot yet distinguish between his physical and emotional internal "things", it must feel a very important matter to decide whether or not it is safe—for himself as well as the recipients—to let his "ins" out: his faeces, but also his feelings, and what he possesses or loves most with the external world.

To do this, he must first learn to trust that his offerings will be respected, welcomed, and not rejected as something "bad". On top of that, he must also assess that giving something up might result in an advantage rather than a deprivation. With regard to his faeces, accordingly, before using the potty a child needs to trust that submitting to the grown-up's request for control will be advantageous not only for others, but for himself as well, affording him greater freedom along with the pleasurable sensation of mastery.

That is the real reason toilet training is such a delicate passage in child development: because it represents the first concrete step towards the possibility of relationships based on *mutual* respect and exchange, rather than a one-sided need to be provided for. Children under three noticeably do not yet know how to play with possessions with each other; fragile and tiny as they are, they appear very "selfish", but not because they are "mean", just because their self-configuration is still, and legitimately, egocentric: needing and expecting to be the "centre of the world". Accordingly, in their view, everything is theirs and they are unwilling to give anything up, to lend one of their games or recognise that someone else's game belongs to him or her. I remember Silvia, the daughter of friends of mine, a little girl not much more than a year old, standing chubby and naked as she looked at the sea in Sardinia. She opened her little arms and exclaimed "Mine!", when even a small wave would have been enough to carry her away.

In conclusion, parents should be patient: any developmental conquest of a new physical ability, such as sphincter control, happens only when it can coincide with the appropriate stage in a child's emotional and cognitive growth.

In the past, preschool started after the age of three and not simply for reasons of hygiene. This is the age when children begin to be able to relate enjoyably and usefully with other children of the same age.

During this gradual acquisition of self-confidence, in this *spontaneous* willingness of the child to move further away from the mother figure to enjoy more complex experiences, parental roles and masculine and feminine templates of care interact naturally in ways similar to those already described in childbirth.

For things to go smoothly, however, we must take into account that the process of moving away from symbiotic primordial security is strongly influenced by the mother's emotional willingness to "let go", to facilitate separation supported by an internal confidence in the new meeting awaiting at every other higher level of complexity and autonomy reached by the child. As in childbirth, the mother is the one who must be emotionally ready for separation and must not feel that the child's attachment to her is a personal belonging she has difficulty giving up. Luckily, here again, as in childbirth, the advantages of growth alleviate the separation, as every step forwards frees the mother from a "layer" of tiring care, but it is fairly easy to try to maintain both advantages and fall into the temptation of keeping possession of a child who has already evolved toward greater autonomy. There is no need for this, as long as one understands and feels that the child's growing process does not hinder the bond between mother and child. On the contrary, as we saw with the transition at the three-month stage, letting go is the condition for the bond to remain unchanged in quality, strength, and intensity, though expressed in ways more suitable to the new age of the child. The archaic and primitive communication must, in fact, be replaced by attitudes and behaviours more appropriate to the evolving relationship. Fear not for the bond: as long as it has been there and has been secure and healthy, a child's attachment to his mother will have the same intensity throughout the child's life; internalised as an inner treasure and model, this will find expression in ever-evolving emotional exchanges. All emotional relationships change over time, but they never decline if their quality and intensity is kept intact.

Whenever mothers have difficulty weaning and blame their children for rejecting separation, if you look more closely you always find that, in reality, it is they, the mothers, who involuntarily and unconsciously refuse to convey the goodness and security of a new acquisition. As if they subtly transmitted that the texture and taste of some good, healthy baby food, for example, was not so great in reality. This invariably happens when a mother, deep inside, harbours a disavowed melancholic longing to keep the baby for herself, so to not be abandoned. When faced with their child's inevitable desire for greater autonomy and separation, such a mother unconsciously fears losing her baby (Phillips, 1999).

The same goes for any protracted habit of sleeping in the parents' bed. When you take the time to listen, you find he is not the real culprit. The fear of separation is, in fact, not only the child's own, but is also mirrored from the mother's or father's emotions (Phillips, 1999).

This is no one's fault; it is just human. We all make mistakes; the important thing is to understand how disadvantageous it can be for everyone, and how much easier and more physiologically acceptable it is to encourage a child's growth by seeking more age-appropriate ways to adequately express this everlasting attachment.

In this regard, I believe that campaigns encouraging breastfeeding should do more to also pass on the emotional significance of this fundamental, but *time-limited* experience. It is not enough to obsessively preach about its importance without also qualifying it as only a step in a slow and constant evolution from the discovery of the relationship to secure autonomy.

However, I would like to stress that weaning is not overcoming a "vice", as might mistakenly be thought. The intensity of the breastfeeding bond must slowly, gradually, be transformed from the initial symbiotic connection through the breast to the possibility of maintaining and expressing attachment differently. This must happen in keeping with the baby's new communication skills, which need to be encouraged so that he can slowly free himself from helpless dependence and reach the stage of desire-driven connection.

By the same token, no protracted breastfeeding can fill the void of separation if a mother is forced by her work obligations into separation too early. I wish all those agencies that promote breastfeeding— including the World Health Organization—would more effectively defend and protect the mother's right to stay close to her baby during his first year of life so that she may fulfil her essential and unique role as nurturer.

The mother figure is not called upon to do all this on her own: this task would be practically superhuman. A woman cannot find in herself alone the resources to simultaneously wean the infant from an attachment which is so strong and also convey that it is safe to go out and conquer the complex reality which the baby must learn to manage in order to become an adult. As in pregnancy and breastfeeding, in fact, the father figure plays a fundamental role in supporting and, ultimately, actively participating in the child's emotional development. Just as the father's voice is perceived indirectly from within the womb during pregnancy, after birth the father figure slowly takes on, as we have seen, a status and role of his own in the child's experience, by distinguishing himself from his initial role as a mummy surrogate. At first, in fact, his role can only adapt to the needs of containment; to cite an example of this only gradual shift from "motherly" to "fatherly" care, you can think of how fathers in neonatal intensive care can effectively alternate with mothers in "kangaroo care". It is so touching to see the newborn, so small and fragile, securely cocooned in the midst of a father's hairy chest. As the child slowly acquires awareness of his own separation and discovers himself as an active interlocutor in the encounters of breastfeeding first and in the relationship later, the figures of mother first and father later begin to take shape in the child's focus. The father, in particular, begins to stand out as a defined character in the emotional affair that unravels from the initial, confused perception.

So, big surprise, the father is not only important for his genetic contribution, he is also an essential player in the child's crucial emancipation from dependency. He is the first loving other outlined on the newborn's horizon, as he is still emotionally one with the maternal figure. From the perspective of the dyad of the symbiotic relationship, he is the third, whom the child will discover and recognise as the preferential interlocutor to go to in his movements away from mother, his trustworthy companion and ally along each step of growth. The father's physical and emotional presence will offer the child the first relational field that is different and alternative from the one with mother: the first discovery of an "other" the child can refer to with trust, the extension of a secure attachment field in the world.

As graphically rendered in the image of the two intersecting sets (Figure 2.1), the father contributes, through his field of experience, to expanding the mother's complementary field of experience, starting from a common emotional area: the one of shared loving care for the child. As we have seen, within this caring matrix the mother supports and encourages the child's separation and exploration further away from herself to a "place" where the father, as in childbirth, welcomes him, supporting his detachment and exploration of the world.

I am very fond of the image depicted in Figure 2.4, and use it here as an example of how a child, still uncertain and full of doubt, looks out to the world through the triangular frame of his father's legs. All tentative, he still needs his dummy between his lips to comfort and remind himself of the continual availability of the maternal field, so difficult to relinquish and where it is so nice to be able to return after an exciting but scary raid out into the world with dad.

However, it is important to recall that even if three-way relationships are happy and pleasant spaces to inhabit, as well as useful and

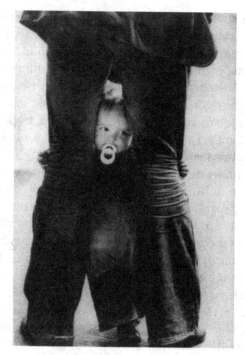

Figure 2.4. Exploring the world with the support of father.

important in the dialectics of quotidian life, it is also fundamental to create boundaries to safeguard the equally important moments of one-to-one interaction.

First of all, the parental couple's intimacy. This in fact, as the baby grows, can and should be gradually recovered and protected. Parents, too, as man and woman, need privacy and physical and emotional intimacy, proof of a passion and complicity that must be kept alive and separate from childcare. The child *will not* mind or be jealous of these moments, as long as he feels loved. Children want their parents to love each other because they can sense the harmony of their affection throughout the household and this reassures them (Winnicott, 1964, 1965a, 1986).

Mother and child's own private moments too should continue and be protected, reconfigured according to the child's growing relational capacities and needs, but never brutally interrupted.

In parallel, it is important to foster father and child's moments: the first thrills of an "accompanied" independence that grants a child the experiences of action and reality testing within a position of security that will increase his self-assurance. I refer here to moments such as when a father and son are busy with household chores, running errands, or carrying out other exploratory activities that often make the child feel proud. Easy evidence of this can be found in children's busy chatter when they come together, often showing off their father, proudly exclaiming "*my* daddy" with an air of feeling untouchable under the protection of a superior being.

Furthermore, the human being is the only animal that creates "culture". This complicates things, because, aside from the development of his natural potential, the individual must also, in order to fit in socially, adapt to and find his or her place within the meaning and value frameworks embodied and enacted within a given society. The father figure is a crucial conveyor of this "creative" adaptation, which should not imply simple subjugation to a set of given rules. The father figure is, in fact, the link between a child's home and the outside world; as mum is on maternity leave, dad will be identified as the one away "working", an expression destined to remain strangely mysterious in the child's mind for a long time. Since this early imprinting, "working" will continue to stand in the child's mind as justification of the fact that the father might be even more absent than the nowadays equally working mother figure. The father's word is also often the last word when it comes to rules.

A "no" from dad, in fact, is much more significant and absolute than the mother's refusal, which the child knows he has more emotional leverage to "sweeten". Very early on, soon after departing from his mother's emotional orbit, the child is confronted with limits and limitations; the first purpose of this is to stop the child harming himself—putting a finger in the electrical socket, burning himself with hot water or the hot iron, or falling down the stairs. Later on, however, limits and rules should acquire the crucial second purpose of setting the boundaries that foster for all of us the possibility to exist and live harmoniously in society, respecting oneself and others and benefiting from the pleasure of interpersonal exchanges and reciprocity.

In setting boundaries, it is useful to be mindful of the fact that a "No", depending on whether it comes from the mother or father, takes on a different flavour for the child. Because the mother's love tends to "contain" (hence the womb as its symbol), the child experiences her "No" as being "held back", kept inside, not allowed to grow and experience life: in other words, the exercise of possession. The father's "No", on the other hand, is experienced by the child as coming from someone who knows his way around in the world. When dad says "No", therefore, he gives the impression of suggesting a route of prudent action and avoidance of danger dictated by his greater experience of the world, rather than an arbitrary limitation of the child's freedom imposed by fear or the mere expression of power.

In Italian, there is an untranslatable term that defines the paternal in a quality quite rare to find nowadays; it could be rendered by "authoritativeness"—as opposed to authoritarianism—referring to that fascinating ability to pass on experience without imposing it. It is a way of pointing to one pathway rather than another, not arbitrarily, but as the outcome of a journey of personal experience and achievement. This stands in contrast to authoritarianism, which is the hysterical imposition of rules set by someone who is only taking advantage of his superior status to humiliate and make those under him suffer what he himself had to undergo when he was an underling. Instead, authoritativeness is more like walking alongside and showing the way, suggesting limits that have been considered and can be explained, accepting mistakes and teaching without anger how to cope with, and navigate, the hardships of life.

The father's role is, therefore, as "sacred", in the sense of its absolute necessity, as the mother's role for the success of the offspring. Creative roles require a good deal of energy and it will be wise to keep a good bit in reserve if one decides to have children (Winnicott, 1988).

If there is one thing that emotionally kills children, it is indifference. It is easier to have a child live through any real difficulty that is recognised, stated, discussed, and shared, than to have him make it through unscathed in an environment of indifference or denial. That is because indifference challenges precisely that basic need every child needs to have met to allow him to grow; the need to transfer his experience into an available adult, to savour its sharing and the ensuing interpersonal meaning-making, so that the outcome of this shared "metabolic" process (with its affective undertones) can be stored inside the child's self like a brick in the building of one's existence, to be used as a framework to deal with similar experiential instances in the future. I remember a sunny afternoon in town as I was walking my dog in the park. I watched a small toddler walking unsteadily, pushing his stroller with his father's help and assailing him with joyous chatter interspersed with incessant interjections and questions. The father was going along absentmindedly, answering now and then with muttering sounds that only made the child come back for more. I was silently suffering. All of a sudden, in front of a dog playground, the child recognised a Dalmatian and ran toward it, shouting "Pongo!"—the name of the lead dog in the Disney film *101 Dalmatians*—as happy as he could be for this authentic emotional encounter (which his dad was not providing, his presence notwithstanding) with the dog. In my heart, I was thankful to Walt Disney for his cartoons.

From childhood dependency to adult reciprocity

Unfortunately, the time we have to raise our children, to make them feel lovingly secure, is limited. It feels long when we are in the midst of it, but, in fact, it flies and it is wise to make the most of it.

A child depends for the most part on his parents until he reaches adolescence, when another major physical and psychological transformation takes place, linked to an important hormonal change that slowly and gradually (once again following the dynamics of childbirth) facilitates the achievement of adult autonomy.

From the age of three all the way up to adolescence, a child becomes more and more able to interact intersubjectively, that is, across difference rather than mere mirroring. He learns how to interact with other people in ways that are gradually less self-centred and with increasing pleasure and curiosity. He comes to appreciate contacts and play with his friends, and his ability for exploration leads him to investigate increasingly complex realities and face new experiences and people with more and more ease. Nevertheless, this widening of experience and know-how that occurs up to adolescence can take place only if fostered and supported by both parents. The child will, in fact, actively and steadily continue to turn to them for reassurance, validation, and the chance to emotionally and cognitively process his own experiences. Imagine a firmly placed compass that draws widening circles, where the relationship between the centre and the opening of the radius is the result of the mediation between the young person's momentum and his parent's loving participation.

The parents' role in this phase has a lot to do with building their child's existential security, not only financially, but, above all, from an emotional point of view. Whether they like it or not, participant or uninvolved, parents always leave a permanent mark on their child's emotional world, whose very landscape will be determined by his childhood experiences. These inevitably form the foundation—shaky or solid, askew or balanced—on which everything else will be built. All experiences, if they are emotionally significant, leave an imprint, but the relationship with one's parents above all others because it is the *first*, and because it has its origin when the infant is totally dependent and relying on his parents to survive. The experience of relatedness with our parents is, therefore, of a different quality with respect to all others as it sets deep, in our somatosensory and emotional memory, the first image of being alive, the first impact and the first flavour of this new path to be trodden and explored. Choosing to ignore this simple, undeniable truth is simply an excuse for dodging the great responsibility that arises from having chosen to reproduce and commit to the demanding task—maybe the most difficult in an individual's life—of good parenting.

However, fatherhood and motherhood imply more than just responsibility, effort, and pain. As we have seen in childbirth, parenthood requires great commitment but offers immense pleasure. It should be enjoyed, not endured. Children can feel and assess quite accurately how much availability and passion underlie their parents' care for them, and this makes an invaluable difference for their future. As human beings are endowed with the imprinting of the womb, with its qualities of holding without compressing, children have an experiential point of comparison to measure the quality of the emotional environment they expect and the one they actually meet.

Parents go from being a protective filter to fundamental emotional reference points to whom the child can confidently take his own experiences to share and process. As he grows older, a child will, in fact, still need, and for a very long time, to be able to count on his parents' availability and to hear their views, especially on salient matters. This will strengthen his identity, widen his competence, and expand his freedom. The birth of any new capacity must be stimulated, recognised, and respected, in a constant, positive encouragement towards taking on those greater responsibilities that come with having "greater powers" as he grows up. Of course, as his growth brings them closer together in age, the relationship between parents and child changes over time. From being protectors, parents gradually become more like companions eventually, albeit without ever losing their role respective to the child. This is safeguarded, in fact, by the presence of an irreconcilable generational gap, which, on the one hand, confers upon the elder party the authoritativeness that comes with greater experience and, on the other hand, inspires respect and gratitude for the loving care and support received.

*   *   *

It is this long emotional experience which unites parents and children from birth through adolescence to adulthood that sets that base of habits, language, beliefs, and values that the child first and the adolescent later will refer to and come to see as essential parts of his own being, the foundation of his identity. The more robust, articulated, shared, talked about, and validated his experiential field can be, the more self-assured and intimately trusting of his own internal references the youth will be in his adolescence. The time between a child is born up until the end of his teenage years is the time for building a solid base, before life carries him away in a whirlwind of complexity—even more so in today's world, despite the apparent simplification of certain aspects of life thanks to technology.

With the arc of an individual's life, adolescence stands out as a second birth, so to speak. It bears all the hallmarks of birth: a physical transformation that marks the passage from one state to another and from one container to the next, accompanied by a slow, gradual, emotional transformation, which overlaps without coinciding with the physical one, and which will take years before becoming fully complete. If childbirth represents the passage from symbiosis to relationship, adolescence marks the passage from family to society. As in childbirth, this transformation is supported by a hormonal modification and, as with childbirth, it is destined to mark, first physically then emotionally, the end of an era. The boundaries of the family environment during this period will no longer be capable of granting satisfaction of the physical, intellectual, and emotional needs of the growing individual. More so than birth, adolescent transformation is generally considered a playground for hormones, as if everything that goes on were almost exclusively a matter of testosterone or oestrogen, and not also, and even more so, a radical emotional development. Yet, this is precisely what adolescence is. Like childbirth, supported by the perfect balance of oxytocin and endorphins, adolescence essentially remains an emotional event. As usual, every reductionist approach that attempts to set aside either the emotional or the physical aspect of what happens is destined, like every simplification, to fail to grasp the real complexity of this period. What was true about childbirth is just as true about adolescence.

During adolescence, first of all a youth really comes into his own "gender," both physically and emotionally. If the distinction between male and female during infancy means little, except for a few propensities usually emphasised by local culture, during adolescence this differentiation not only occurs, but begins to take on full significance. Sexual development not only means a new sensitivity to the physical and emotional difference between the genders, but it entails that slow, gradual transformation in the way we want to express love and to whom which underlies sexual encounters. However, it is not only that: coming to sexual maturity also entails the development of new, gender-diverse ways of responding to the needs of life.

I am personally convinced that the reason for love, for its existence and necessity, lies in the existence of limitations. If we had no limits, if we could be completely self-sufficient and all-entailed from an evolutionary standpoint, we would not need to love each other. A parent's love warmly envelopes the needy, helpless baby. The relationship is uneven, asymmetric. The child has only needs; he cannot give; he is in need of a selfless love, but cannot respond to this except by showing his gratification. Motherhood and fatherhood have within them this generous willingness, this capability to feel repaid just by the well-being and, later, the gratitude on the part of a child who has been adequately cared for. Therefore, the limit that "justifies" and gives foundations to the parent–child relationship is the child's helplessness: the little one in need of the big one, the fragile in need of the strong, the unknowing in need of the knowing. This is an uneven, asymmetrical relationship that changes over time, as the child grows and becomes more capable of exchanges, but the asymmetry can never be completely smoothed out because of the generational gap.

Building on the foundations of childhood, the individual as his own or her own person is gradually formed during adolescence. It is now that the function of limit serving the search for love and for a love partner takes a different direction. Indeed, sexual determination into male or female creates a biological limit to the individual, on the basis of the fact that he or she is (for the great majority) physically limited to belonging to one gender only and not the other one. Secondary sexual characteristics all of a sudden appear and make their differences clearly visible to these former children. So troubling, yet awaited, is this determination—with the same anxiety that comes physiologically with every change—that both male and female teenagers initially tend to gather into gender-based groups, in search for the security of *sameness*, while casting inquisitive looks upon the *others*, the ones different from one's self. Teenage cliques can, therefore, be seen as naïve, rather sweet, forms of identity defence. The big change here is that this suddenly attractive "other" is not a "grown-up". The object of desire is an equal to one's self, yet different at the same time. The irresistible call, the ground-breaking transformation that is sparked by adolescence, is that, for the first time, it is not need, but curiosity, desire, and choice that constitute the drives to form attachments. Whereas, during infancy a child looks onto the world mainly in need of care due to his fragility and helplessness, an adolescent looks upon life with desire: he is driven to what attracts him, fascinates him, what awakes his curiosity. He starts looking for the other-than-self, not out of necessity but desire; this shift does not only involve sexuality—still tentative and in need of a slow reinforcement—but it encompasses the whole approach to life. During adolescence, we see the beginning of an emotional transformation, supported by a physical one, which, over the years, will shift gratification from the realm of need—where the provider cannot be chosen—to desire, which, instead, requires, to be secure, discrimination and choice of referents.

Therefore, if newborns need their carer to provide the protection and containment lost at childbirth, adolescents—even though still uncertain of their identity, values, status, and opinions—search the realm of life for travel companions with whom to grow and share views, games, and passions. Great friendships are made during adolescence, a time when, without severing the strong ties to parents and family, the impetuous, irresistible urge is felt to be free, to make daring personal choices, and to play by one's own rules.

Motivation supporting attachment needs also changes in adolescence. Love moves from a level where the attachment figure is needed as a support to provide security towards a meeting of two individuals—complete in their identity, limited in their differences—who travel together the path of life out of *mutual choice*. Naturally, it will take years for such a transformation to take place. Every phase of development has its specific goals to reach within a certain time frame, but every subsequent step—as it increases in complexity—requires more time to be fully achieved. So, if developmental goals took hours in childbirth and months of internalisation in childhood, the passages that will take an individual from adolescence to adulthood turn into years to complete. As we have seen, in fact, nature proceeds in leaps and bounds that require long periods of latency, preparation, and processing.

During adolescence, the original family never disappears, but, in a certain sense, it shifts its centre, moving to support the adolescent from behind the scenes. The honour of centre stage should, in fact, be entrusted to the youth, as parents lovingly and trustingly move into the background, behind the curtains, still capable of watchful participation or suggestions when required.

Still, during this transformation, the mother and father's gaze— with their respective meanings—is of great value in facilitating and accompanying the change and consolidation of their child's forming identity. I am thinking of the powerful validation inherent in, for example, the father's look of ecstatic admiration (remember the peasant-hunter in Giorgione's picture) as he observes the transformation of his little girl into an attractive woman; or, how a mother can be deeply and proudly moved as she sees her boy grow into a man and an appealing partner for another woman; for the teenager, these are the earliest validations and confirmations of the ongoing development towards the achievement of an identity as man or woman which is still in the making and foggy, but which he or she can feel is supported and cherished by the parents' emotional participation.

Nowadays, however, parental involvement in childcare tends, sadly, to be upside down. It is very easy, in fact, for the child to be left to his own devices at an early age, out of ignorance of his needs and of how human development takes place, with the presumption that he cannot understand anyway who is there and who is not, and that he needs very little. Then, when he becomes an adolescent and should be let go (though within boundaries appropriate to his age), the tendency is to block him off, to keep him under undermining control for fear of his new and greater contact with the world at large and the dangers it hides. This kind of behaviour is totally opposite to Winnicott's evocative image of the parenting trajectory from a presence capable of maintaining the "initial illusion" to facilitating and allowing a gradual "disillusion": that is, the encounter with reality and confrontation with life as the child grows into a youth and then an adult.

If we, as parents, still want to protect our teenage children from the harshness of life or the false allures of a dangerous society, prohibitions and constrictions are useless. Actually, the only real antidote lies in the parents' ability to build, in the intimacy of their relationship with the adolescent, a strong attachment and identity model alternative to the ones proposed by the false idols to which he or she will inevitably be exposed. An embodied example of adult life made of the shared experiences of love, passion, commitment, and the acceptance that exertion and even pain sometimes are the necessary means through which true happiness, well-being, and achievements can be obtained.

Although these modelling experiences are strengthened during adolescence, they begin earlier, right from childhood, provided the child has enjoyed an emotional environment where feelings—both positive and negative—are accepted, known, shared, and protected. An environment where both attachment and individuation needs and their related emotions are cherished as sacred: the very keepers of the truth and pleasure of life. Once you have breathed in a healthy "emotional field", it is hard to lose its imprinting, and not discriminate it from the false temptations one is exposed to. I say, provocatively, that a teenager who has been brought up on healthy home-cooking might submit to McDonald's to please the group, but will hold on to the memory of a good meal and try to get back to one as soon as possible.

Post-adolescent mature attachment, therefore, finds its prerequisite in emotional self-awareness, slowly built through the years of availability, mirroring, and validation in the family. Knowledge and acceptance of one's needs, limits, and desires can now be translated into the ability to orientate oneself in life to find relational environments capable of meeting them and wishing to be met in turn. As opposed to the young child, in fact, as we grow into adulthood we need and want not only to be recipients, but providers too, to be part of a reciprocal exchange of mutual and irreplaceable choice. The awareness of one's needs is, therefore, paired with an equal awareness of one's own creative and emotional endowment in search of relationships in which to express itself.

This is the physiological evolution of the child's needs for both attachment and exploration, security and creative play: the same necessities expressed at a higher level of complexity and reciprocity in the well-adjusted adult. The youth shall then need, on the one hand, to find a professional pathway capable of providing him with creative fulfilment and a sense of usefulness, as something that allows him to express himself and his abilities, and, on the other hand, listen to his need for loving bonds capable of replacing and expanding upon the family reference. Not only romantic love, therefore, but a network of relations providing a sense of belonging and of not being alone. This, and this only, can recreate that wonderful feeling of security experienced in the early attachments: a sense of being accompanied in one's existence by others who are capable of sharing our joys and difficulties; attachment figures who are now valued for their difference from us, yet found similar in the sharing of the human condition with its vulnerability to solitude and fear.

This template finds its ultimate actualisation in adult romantic love between two partners who finally find in each other their chosen companion. A bond no longer based on dependence, but on exchange. A bond that is heir to the early infantile need for asymmetrical love, but is now made of complicity, sharing, passion, and attraction. An adult reciprocity, then, which should be established as the mature fulfilment of human emotionality, able to trigger the release of those same endorphins underpinning our species' sense of security just as the mother–child relationship did at the start of life, as pointed out by neurobiology.

Nature has awarded adult romantic relationships with the ability to reproduce. Procreation is not contemplated before adolescence for the simple reason that the option is not available to children because they are too busy growing up themselves. Adult sexuality should, therefore, come equipped with an adequate emotional maturity, one that includes the ability to love, share, and take responsibility.

If, for a child, growing up is a difficult though thrilling undertaking, then bearing the responsibilities of adult life is just as demanding for an adult. If he is aware of this and accepts his human limits, an adult should allow himself time to refuel, to take physical and emotional breaks in order to prevent what is nowadays called "stress" from gnawing at him in the rush and tension of his daily concerns. The adolescent transformation, in fact, does not equal an erasure of our childhood needs, it just entails that as adults we can be our own direct referents instead of passing through parents to be able to bring our needs and wishes to the world of life to be met. Just as our adult features keep some remnants of our childhood body, so, too, does our emotional "inner child", so to speak, stay on within our adulthood: the phases and needs of childhood are never overcome, they are integrated into adulthood. Adult life runs not only along the tracks of ability and efficiency. On the contrary, the perception and respect of one's inner child must be preserved. We still need nourishment when we grow up; we just change the way we obtain it. We go from breastfeeding to baby food then on to acquiring and cooking it ourselves, but the basic need is the same: hunger. The same happens with love: the modalities and how we love changes, but the need for love and affection remains, ineluctable because it is part of human nature (Suttie, 2014).

Therefore, during adult life there is, or should be, an alternation between moments of creative ability and productivity on the one hand, and on the other special moments of regression that allow us to relax, pamper ourselves, and become "little" again, just for a little while. Not only childbirth, but also life itself, should be an alternating succession of moments of effort and moments of peaceful surrender and release. For example, sleep is a fundamental source of recovery. During sleep, one can forget everything while resting and going back to being "little" in surrendering to dreams with trusting abandon, "tucked in" between the sheets while one's emotional life expresses itself free of any scruples or impediments. Those whose sleep is disturbed by nagging thoughts about their daytime worries will actually not be able to "turn off" and take full advantage of the restorative pause to regain strength. By alternating daytime and night-time, nature teaches and facilitates a balance between work and rest, making it almost compulsory to stop what one is doing at sunset in the wilderness. Instead, in our modern city lives, with lights on at every hour, natural rhythms are easy to ignore, and we forget that these limits are not just physical and astronomical, but also have significance for our emotional needs.

There are various, indeed innumerable, ways to "turn off", rest, relax, and recuperate. I think of walks in the park, the pleasure of sports, watching a beautiful sunset or a starry sky when we are lucky enough to catch a glimpse of one. I think of the pleasures of friendship, the joy of meeting up with someone and sharing emotions as well as worries, of doing things together, or just chatting. I think of music, how close it can be to our own feelings, sometimes playful, sometimes tragic or sentimental; I am thinking of how it can bring people together, give a feeling of belonging, of something to share; I am thinking also of how easily music can suggest the perception of the limit, and, therefore, of what is transcendent. I think of political passions, of the strength of ideals that drives us to overcome the limited experience of the present by imagining the possibility of a better future world. I think of the various expressions of culture, literature, theatre, cinema, and art, which contribute to placing our existence in a historical continuum capable of going beyond our individual existence, projecting us into a mysterious and infinite dimension through our connection and participation to a collective narrative.

It is easy to observe how the voracious market forces of our society have cast their nets over all of these fundamental expressions of the beauty of human experience; we should not be deterred, however, as beneath the vulgar exploitation, true values remain unchanged.

Finally, I mention sexuality, obviously not as merchandise or as a quick and uncommitted corollary to a lifetime measured in terms of consumption and appropriation. On the opposite end of the spectrum, I am not referring either to "sexuality as it ought to be", but simply meaning to describe it as it really is, in its essence and natural meaning.

Sexual intercourse is, in fact, an encounter, the most profound one, which, in adulthood, reproduces and even surpasses the baby's experience of loving unity with his mother's body, transfiguring it and making it the place of fertility. Indeed, of all these innumerable ways to "turn off" and recharge that I have mentioned above, and which we should joyfully offer ourselves alternated with a serious and responsible participation in life, sexuality is, for its physical and emotional nature, what most resembles and reproduces the symbiotic fusion and secure surrender we all experienced in our mother's womb. This even more than sleep itself, because it is relational.

Through choice and desire, in sexuality there is, in fact, a search for the "other" with whom to practise and saturate our fundamental need for physical bonding and tenderness, a need which accompanies us—encrypted in our corporeity—throughout our lives, well beyond childhood. In the physical and emotional fusion of sexuality, two bodies physically become one, as they were at the beginning of life, merging in an embrace and the trusting abandonment of orgasm. If well lived, sexuality can, through reciprocity and exchange, evoke that same magical unity that gave meaning to the beginning, that same joy of feeling loved and accepted which so deeply governs our whole existence.

One last remark: even in the fusion of bodies, emotions, and minds that characterises intercourse, masculine and feminine templates remain distinct and complement each other. This is because sexual development runs along a different pathway in males and females. In their early years, both little girls and boys start off from a position of deep, preferential attachment to their mother's body because it represents their origin, where they came from. Body contact with mother symbolises and evokes primeval security, protection. So, children of either gender are obviously strongly dependent on the mother's body, and, to be able to grow, both need to slowly separate themselves from *her* body. Not the father's for girls and the mother's for boys: the longed-for primary object to find security is the maternal one for both.

During adolescence, a girl, who will already have lovingly toyed with her own future maternal role through her play, suddenly finds herself in the midst of a major physical transformation that will slowly bring her body to assume more and more the likeness of her beloved mother's figure. With surprise and wonder, she will look at herself in the mirror and see, from the incipient curves her body is taking, that the miracle has occurred; she has become the mother; she has her features; the object of her love becomes her physical and emotional likeness. I remember something the eldest of my daughters told me when, in her early puberty, her physical changes were just starting to take shape. She came to me one day in a thoughtful mood and said, "You know, mummy, I get it; we're the stars and they're the planets that circle around us." I couldn't but confirm her words.

Indeed, I believe there is a natural central positioning, a sacredness linked to the biological maternal role, which bestows a particular emotional resonance upon the female figure, not only to men but to all human beings who came from a woman's womb. Think of the early terracotta figures of Mother Earth and fertility goddesses. This is not a matter of superiority, just the highly symbolic quality of the female body's function: its ability to give life, which, however, would not be possible if not met by a man's desire. I find here again a sense of total balance, exactly thanks to the differences.

From the very start, unknowingly extraneous and intrinsically different from the maternal body which he comes from and depends upon, during adolescence the boy undergoes a physical transformation which differentiates him even more from the longed-for object. In the teenage years, his body gets stronger and grows hair, his voice becomes manly and deep, and he discovers himself more and more different and separate from that loved feminine body. This, in turn, becomes a set goal to re-conquer: not any more in a dependent infantile modality, but with the joy and pride of being able to become for a woman, as father has been for mother, that loving presence which can make her so beautiful, so attractive, and capable of giving heterosexual life.

This symbolical significance contributes to giving human sexuality a profound and precious value, as it links it with the critical issues of trust and surrender, independently from procreation. In sexual intercourse, the male can actually re-enter the female body to find again, through pleasure, that primal belonging which fortifies and soothes him; the woman complementarily embraces, experiencing a pleasure that goes hand in hand with her capacity to open and contain—something not too far away, emotionally, from the maternal. The sexual hormones are, once again, oxytocin and endorphins.

The actualisation of this complementarity, the attainment of this balanced relatedness, lies at the foundations of the possibility of bringing new creatures to life, creatures who, in turn, will hopefully be able one day to make once again this compelling encounter between male and female the secure base for starting a new life and extending the horizon of our species across time.

Therefore, in adult life, attachment and emotions continue to play a fundamental role for us to be able to find meaning in our existence, striving both towards the expression of, and delight in, our capacities—our very own talents—and towards the building and maintaining of a sound relational life. The more our need for attachment and relatedness is recognised and responded to during infancy and childhood, the more in adulthood one will be able to recognise these needs (as they will be referenced to the experience of having them met in childhood), respect them, and take agency to find someone capable and wishing to meet them again, thereby finding well-being and fulfilment.

* * *

For a long time, science and philosophy have reprehensibly disregarded the emotional and attachment components making up human nature, whereas only recently they have been understood in their fundamental importance to our very survival. When considering issues of health, at both the individual and societal levels, we must begin to encompass the necessity for a new cultural respect for our core attachment and emotional needs. I believe that only starting from this premise we may draw inspiration towards a transformation of the current social and cultural establishment in the direction of creating a human environment capable of meeting the demands of our nature. An attachment-based understanding of our existence tells us how important the emotional roots of our being are, as they lie at the foundations of our well-being and happiness, both in childhood and adult life. We need a society that takes this into account and makes it its priority to respect and forge the fulfilment of our attachment and emotional needs.

Note

1. Estivill and a co-author have also published a manual extending his sleep method "to make children eat" (Estivill & Domènech, 2005). I would argue, ironically, that parenting would be a superhuman task if we were really to make up for, and actively teach, basic fundamental autonomic responses which, according to Estivill, nature would have failed to pass on. In opposition to Estivill and Domènech, see Juul (2001) on the "competent" baby.

CHAPTER THREE

The need for a cultural revolution

I f our emotional life is so important for our survival and so deeply ingrained in our physical and biological make-up, then the spontaneous question which comes to mind is: how could Western scientific thought have neglected it so thoroughly? How could it be so utterly ignored until only very recently?

Whenever I discuss our emotional world, I always have the feeling I am referring to something that is mostly taken for granted, but which in fact has barely been studied in any depth and, therefore, remains little known. Even though the study of emotions has a sound scientific basis, I find that it is either underestimated as a subject matter everyone is superficially but adequately proficient in, or else it is delegated to "specialists" who usually express themselves so cryptically and with such incomprehensible terminology that everyone concludes it is something too complex to be explained to the layman, let alone understood.

In such a current state of things, it is, therefore, unlikely that any consideration of our fundamental emotional needs may come into play within the public discussion of issues such as the economy, the environment, employment, social (in)security, inequality, development, war or peace. It seems paradoxical, but the truth is that even a culture like ours, whose greatest pride lies in its scientific knowledge and resources, has only recently begun to apply science to affectivity. It is only in the past century, in fact that the West has come to understand and theorise the importance and centrality of emotional bonds and to investigate them further from a scientific point of view.

The first studies on the subject appeared only in the 1950s, as great authors such as Spitz, Bowlby, Winnicott, and Mahler began to take note of and investigate the effects of deprivation on war orphans and other abandoned children. These very studies were so groundbreaking in the truths they unearthed that they imprinted a U-turn on the development of psychoanalytical thought as well as of therapeutic techniques forever after. More recently, modern neurobiology and research with ultrasound scanners have confirmed both the importance and the early development of emotional bonds. They have also clarified the central role attachment plays in the physical and emotional survival of our species and underlined the crucial influence early attachment has on individual development. Studies in ethnology and anthropology have also confirmed the innate preparedness and prevalence of prosocial instincts such as maternal preoccupation, empathy, caring behaviour, and solidarity, understanding them as *emerging factors*[1] in human evolution—factors that have guaranteed our survival as a species, let alone a degree of quality of life (Bertirotti, 2008, 2009; de Waal, 1996; Tinbergen, 1951; also see *La Repubblica*, 2007).

All this notwithstanding, it remains bewildering how the currently available scientific knowledge of the psychological and cognitive developmental process which, supported and facilitated by the presence of good-enough parental figures, renders the transformation possible from the infant's primary total dependence to the slow and gradual conquest of autonomy in adult individuals of our species—a developmental process currently understood as an essential condition for physical and emotional health—mostly remains a little known truth. Even progressive campaigns such as the ones encouraging natural birthing, "rooming in" (letting the newborn stay in the same hospital room as his mother, as opposed to taking him to the nursery), or breastfeeding, tend to focus exclusively on a partial objective. What I think would be more incisive would be a more general form of campaigning, one centred on a reconsideration of the human dimension through and through. This, in fact, could defend the centrality of every person's emotional development from the basis of sound

scientific premises, rather than a somewhat vague romantic senti-
mentalism, and, therefore, have more leverage to be heard, spread
awareness, and raise a collective commitment to create serious
measures to safeguard and foster those conditions that are necessary
for the healthy emotional development of our children.

We witness instead a concerning delay in giving any serious
consideration to the relational aspects that foster our existence, aside
from calling on the "mental hygiene experts" to manage and contain
the growing number of people suffering from psychological disturbances arising from the contradictions of our way of life, where the
implicit message is to identify the sufferers and quickly and efficiently
normalise them so they can go back to being producers and consumers. I believe that such a collective depreciation still assigned to all
things "emotional" is a manifestation of the profound, subterranean
influence that Western philosophical and scientific tradition still holds
over our thought and, thereby, over our social organisation and system
of values. This tradition has, in fact, historically been incapable of
reconciling body and mind in one single hypothesis respectful of the
complexity of living beings, and has thereby for a long time failed to
understand the place of Man in relation to nature. A nature, both
within and without, which inherently and obviously conditions us, but
which at the same time clearly indicates what should be done to direct
evolution and growth—not only in the sense of maximising utility—
towards useful objectives which may safeguard and facilitate our
survival.

More specifically, when I mention Western scientific thought here,
I am referring to its Galilean–Newtonian roots, something we learn to
take for granted from our studies as if it were a fully adequate,
unquestionable explanation of reality. An "absolute", existing outside
time and history, when, instead, its heuristic power has long been
questioned, at least in science itself.

A brief plunge into the history of philosophy

Before I proceed any further with my reflections, I feel a small digres-
sion on this matter is necessary. I believe, in fact, that any attempt to
work towards a greater understanding of human beings, to be of any
value, must start from an acknowledgement of the biases affecting the

idea of Man that we have inherited from our culture—an image we are presently struggling with as the severity of the threat to our very survival on planet earth is forcing us to rethink the organisation of our society. As for any other human construction, the idea of Man that a society holds is informed by a culturally specific outlook on reality. In the West, we find that, since the late sixteenth century, every product of thought has been strongly influenced by the (indiscriminate) application of a scientific framework which was actually developed to interpret a *specific* and *limited* area of reality: specifically, inert objects in a void. However, the level of meaning-making extrapolated by the experimental method has instead seen its use unduly expanded to interpret the complexities of nature and life, which require, as we shall see, quite a different set of tools for their interpretation and understanding.

Working as a therapist alongside doctors and nurses, in both psychiatric and maternity wards, I have had many an opportunity to conflict with their objectifying, medical attitude towards patients. However, I abandoned any confrontational stance towards them as soon as I realised that their studies and preparation had actually hindered them from any temptation to move past a strictly objectivist point of view. It was not their ignorance, but their very "expertise" which imposed on them an exclusive focus on the evaluation of symptoms. Only patient, daily association with them, and my encouragement to assume a different perspective, would eventually have the effect of drawing the medical staff I worked alongside with into a broader consideration of the "case".

As we have introduced earlier, the development of medicine, biology, anthropology, sociology, and economics, as well as psychology, and, in general, of all the so-called humanities, was influenced by the philosophical underpinnings at the basis of the method of the "exact physical sciences", which was born with Galileo at the end of the sixteenth century. Since then, all the sciences, if they wanted to be deemed as such, were implicitly forced to embrace a method which would prove completely ineffective in accounting for the phenomena under scrutiny in domains where complexity reigns.

This clarification is particularly important to me because, as a clinician, I believe progress towards change, be it personal or collective, cannot be made without an understanding of any biasing legacy that has to be worked-through—patiently and with no pointless recriminations or blame.

As for me, I learnt early on to doubt scientific "certainties". Even as an adolescent, and before entering my philosophical and scientific studies, I remember struggling to understand why my experience of life—with its wealth of feelings and complexity of thoughts—seemed poorly represented in the categories proposed by the adults who surrounded and instructed me. Later, I had the good fortune of meeting great mentors who would guide me towards a way of thinking that would instead appease my doubts and stimulate my creativity. To this day, in looking back, I consider my university studies fundamental tools in my thought processes, still valuable in supporting and informing my overall view on life; in particular, I feel that having the chance, during my studies in philosophy, to delve deeper into the origins and history of Western scientific thought is what has afforded me greater freedom than most in moving beyond explored and pre-established patterns.

In the 1960s, I found myself struggling (as I still do) with the lingering in science of what I would eventually recognise as an outdated, nineteenth century framework, still based on determinism and reductionism. This mindset, moreover, I then noticed prevailed not only in science but also (alas!) in everyday attitudes. Already then, such an approach appeared to me inexplicably superficial, and significantly unable—or, as I would now say, unwilling—to reflect on the complex and dramatic events that had just occurred during the war, as well as on the great changes taking place in society.

Despite its inefficacy, however, this reductionist way of thinking seems not to have shifted in the subsequent forty years, but still prevails. It can be recognised, for instance, in what appears to be a general urgency to turn the page, to forget the tragedies and suffering, burying memory under the myth of wealth and superficial hedonism, the so-called consumer society. Thus, small luxuries, justified in the 1940s and 1950s after so much suffering, slowly became vices. False needs and freedoms were sold to us as the modern achievements of civilisation, presented as progress but really incapable of giving any true satisfaction or gratification.

For this reason, I would argue that the 1960s and 1970s debate questioning the dominant way of thought and denouncing its inability to comprehend and explain the limits and defects of our current lifestyle is sadly very much still relevant today. Similarly, I still find dramatically contemporary the criticism of then denouncing a mentality of avoidance of problems and responsibilities which had come to prevail with the advent of consumerism.

Therefore, I thought that it might be useful to provide a brief overview here of what my mentors taught me to see, in the belief that their words—still a source of great inspiration and awe for me—in reaching those who have not been lucky enough to meet them or read any of their works, may help us shed some light on the issues we are still grappling with today. I intend the following considerations as useful tools, not in any way meant to question or argue in favour of tossing out our entire culture, but simply as means to reflect upon it. Only by investigating the roots and biases of our culture, in fact, I believe that we may be able to better understand why it is so difficult, even today, for us to shift to more appropriate methods to identify and solve the problems that surround us, problems we would like to overcome. I also hope that the following might inspire and convince the reader, as it persuaded me back then, of the necessity of integrating methods and insights coming from many disciplines when the subject of enquiry is human beings, what secures our survival, and what makes us happy. This, if we want our findings to provide a faithful and respectful account of the complexity that qualifies our species.

Joseph Needham: a scientist who reconsidered Western scientific premises through the eyes of another culture

In the course of my studies in philosophy, my encounter with the works of Joseph Needham was to guide me through an in-depth investigation into the origins of Western scientific thought, a research aimed at identifying its peculiarities and originality as well as its limits. Through his work, I discovered that science, in that Galilean–Newtonian form that reigned throughout the nineteenth century, has, in fact, been a limited phenomenon. I learnt that this particular method for the creation and organisation of knowledge was created in a given place and under specific circumstances, and that it is neither the only method nor the only framework that mankind has ever devised to approach the study of nature. I thereby learnt that it is not an absolute standard, but a valid instrument of enquiry only under certain circumstances. To use a metaphor, even if one cannot make an entire dress out of a handkerchief, the handkerchief is still useful in its own domain. However, other cultures have organised their thought and scientific theories differently.

I believe that Needham's thought is still an extraordinary inspiration for this sort of reflection. Born in England in 1900, Joseph Needham trained as a biologist to then specialise in the biochemistry of embryonic development, but alongside his field of expertise he had also always had a deep interest in the philosophical underpinnings of science. At Cambridge in the 1930s—along with great scientists such as Bernal, Bateson, Bragg, and Rutherford—Needham became involved in the then lively dispute between supporters of mechanism and vitalism. Even at the beginning of the twentieth century, conflict in fact already existed between supporters of the theory that, in the wake of Galileo and Newton, argued that Nature could be conceived as a great machine in which all phenomena, including biological ones, were explainable in purely physical and mechanical terms, and others who instead favoured a spiritualistic approach that attributed more than purely physical and chemical characteristics to the phenomena of life.

Refusing to align with either side in this age-old dispute, Needham favoured a more original stance aimed at overcoming "the insoluble enigma of object and subject" or, as he later defined it, the "Western neurosis of the separation between matter and spirit".

He argued that, as human investigators of nature, objective as we may well aspire to be, we still cannot but start from that cluster of sensations that is always present within us, accompanying our experience of being throughout our entire life. We cannot, in fact, free ourselves from our physical body because it is always with us, "forming a more or less prominent feature in the flow of our thoughts and feelings" (Needham, 1925, p. 256). As an embryologist, Needham alluded to the complex physical–emotional unit which is the make-up of human beings and advocated the need for us to understand this unit in its original and extraordinary oneness, resisting the temptation of splitting it in two or flattening it into one-sided interpretations so to conform to the standard imposed by the positive sciences.

This was all very contemporary, as, at the beginning of the past century, the scientific community was forced to confront an age-old dilemma, which had already risen to the fore again and again in the history of Western thought, but never been resolved: namely, the separation of mind and body, the compartmentalisation of spirit and matter into two ironclad domains created to solve the troubling issue opened by Galileo. It so happened in fact that, in eventually having to recognise the indisputable truth of the evidence regarding the earth's movement around the sun, the Catholic Church had to reverse itself and recognise some value of truth to science. Therefore, it "settled" the dilemma by giving science free reign, or at least a freer reign, over matter, while still maintaining its authority over the spiritual realm. Thus, the two sides were separated, even opposed, making it for a long time difficult, if not impossible, to have any meaningful discussion capable of bringing together what had been split.

In considering whether a scientific method capable of accounting for the complexity of reality could be found, Needham came to the conclusion that the abstract mathematical world, founded on logic, induction, and statistics, could not be considered an adequate tool, since it can only offer an essentially intellectual, metric description of the living world. By taking this position, Needham, while upholding the relative validity of scientific interpretations of reality, also underlined its limits and rebelled against what he saw as an inappropriate extension of a mechanistic mentality to the exploration of complex phenomena, such as the ones of biological or human and social nature.

> The universe of science is a construct of our imagination; it is deterministic, but we unconsciously reject what would make it different. It is ordered, but we select, from the infinite number of facts, facts to put in order. It is rational, but we are too, and we render it such. (Needham, 1929, p. 66)

Heisenberg would later say, "Natural science, does not simply describe and explain nature; it is part of the interplay between nature and ourselves" (Heisenberg, 1958, p. 81). In other words, Man unavoidably intervenes with his own intellectual activity—inevitably influenced by culture—in organising knowledge according to historically defined categories and values.

My quote from Heisenberg is not accidental, as it was exactly the new theories emerging at Needham's time in physics, such as Heisenberg's indetermination principle, Einstein's theory of relativity, and the development of quantum mechanics, that most incontrovertibly showed how the classic methods of interpreting natural phenomena were proving insufficient in describing an unforeseen complexity lying at the very core of matter and its dynamics.

In the same way that these new areas of investigation found the classic framework of Western science lacking, so would the phenomenon of life. Biology appeared problematic because, as Needham pointed out, we do not possess a category of interpretation of reality capable of linking the living with the non-living. This does not mean necessarily that such a link does not exist in nature—it might—but, in the development of our culture, we have not been able to turn the evidence of a link into a category that would allow us to see it, as we have founded our knowledge on the postulate of an inherent discontinuity between matter and spirit. This split between body and mind, matter and spirit, is, however, just a culturally specific historical product, occurring over a long period of time as the result of specific events in the philosophy of science. Nevertheless, a pertinacious failure or unwillingness to consider the interdependency of the two domains, which resulted in an unfaltering blind reliance on inadequate methods of appraising and making sense of reality, is, unfortunately, not limited to the world of science. Our everyday lives, our most common gestures, and the decisions we make in all matters appear in fact to be influenced by a "popular version" of the prototypical scientist's mindset—with its hidden baggage of postulates, pseudo-certainties, subsidiary beliefs, and convictions.

This way, the roots of Man, which in the past were well-rooted in the earth, are now isolated by layers of steel, glass, and concrete from any living contact with this. And let us not fool ourselves that this process has almost arrived at a conclusion; on the contrary the future holds nothing but a long series of pseudo-triumphs, further acquisition of power over nature, and further temptation to sever every living connection with this. (Needham, 1931, p. 14)

The good news is that, clearly, if the opposition between mind and body, or matter and spirit, has a historical origin, it can be surmounted.

The modern ideal of mathematical science was brought to light in mechanics through Newton's *Principi*. Thus it was quite natural to take mathematics as the perfect example of scientific systematization, both present and future. It was supposed that other sciences would have developed, not merely as mechanics, but as special chapters of mechanics. Until the end of the last century, it was universally assumed that all natural movements could one day be referred to the equations of classical mechanics. But today we know that not only can sociology not be referred to mechanics through biology and physics, but also that physics itself could not be conformed to this artificial model. Neither electrodynamics, nor atomic physics, nor quantum theory can be derived from the principals of classical mechanics. (Needham, 1968, p. 25)

If scepticism means not believing that a single specific field of experience is capable of providing an exhaustive vision of reality, then Needham professed himself a sceptic. He argued that a scientist needs history, philosophy, psychology, and spirituality in order to escape the invisible, but steel-strong, cage of his intellectual pride and be able to re-establish contact with the social human world. The same goes for the historian, philosopher, psychologist, or poet. Ethics, then, becomes the awareness that the world is a whole of which mankind is an active part.

Biological order is, therefore, different from the order we find in physics or chemistry, but this does not mean that there is no order, or that the human mind cannot penetrate it. It is a question of finding new concepts, such as "field" or "organisation", and postulating that what appears to be qualitatively different derives from the very properties of the elements that make it up, properties that, however, become actualised only in relation to specific states of complexity.

If his criticism of the reigning scientism brought Needham the biologist closer to organicism, as a philosopher his encounter with dialectic materialism and Marxism introduced him to the analysis of the dynamics reigning the collective dimension of human existence. The integration of these two pathways of investigation brought Needham to a philosophical synthesis in which his organicism, now definitely freed from transcendence, would include ethics and politics in an evolutionary vision of nature's becoming.

In this vision, good no longer needs a supernatural basis. It is, instead, a natural category of organisation, posed to emerge and be realised at the adequate level of complexity. Thereby, the very sense of the *numinous*, the sacred indissolubly tied to ethics, which Needham had strenuously defended against the dogmatic pretences of science, is transferred back onto earth and becomes *social emotion*. "The sacred is far from being the 'wholly other'; it is the quality of the secular raised to its highest power and consecrated to the noblest purposes" (Needham, 1945, p. 120). In other words, Man, as an integral part of nature, plays an active part in it. Our minds and feelings are not discontinued from nature, something apart, but, on the contrary, we take part in the natural dynamic—already begun at the biological level—that tends towards the gradual organisation of reality towards greater complexity. Through trials and errors, advancements and reversals, mankind in Needham's view irresistibly moves towards the best organisation possible for the survival of all its members, towards a happier and a freer form of life for all. To speak of the inevitability of society's evolution in these terms has nothing teleological, but simply means to affirm scientifically how the presence of contradictions necessarily leads to the search for, and realisation of, a way out. This is not about abstractly discussing evil in the world. It is, instead, about intervening in the world to correct it.

Needham, however, warns that this process does not occur mechanically or passively, but through the work of Man. Taking responsibility over our being an active part of this dynamic in fact implies not only a transformation of social structures, but also a reclamation of our humanity, a process that needs to take place in every one of us. It is about rediscovering oneself, rediscovering one's own nature, one's own human aspirations buried under a civilisation that has done so much for mankind's dominion over Nature as to forget Man as her subject.

As far back as 1936, in *The Biological Basis of Sociology*, Needham stated the need for a form of mental health, which, by identifying and analysing states of mental distortion such as neurosis, paranoia, and sadism, would eventually be able to point as to the conditions that allow for human beings to fully realise their humanity. "I believe the movement started by Freud to have implications of greater sociological importance than many have stated until now" (Needham, 1945, p. 160). Needham also wonders why a new concern for mental well-being only arose so late in history. His answer was because the more free we become from the shackles of our material needs, the more easily and successfully we have the resources to move towards the "good". However, in such a quest for realising our full humanity, material wealth remains useless, unless we also liberate ourselves from the conditioning of the false assumptions and prejudices of a cultural heritage that actually hinders and prevents us from becoming realised in harmony with our own nature. The search for the "good", from this perspective, therefore becomes an asymptotic longing for and tending to, which preserves and does not need to discount the sense of the numinous, itself born out of the very limits and mystery that accompany the life of everyone.

So, the idea of Man as a machine was replaced in Needham's thought by a concept of the human being as an organism that is intelligent and sensitive to emotions, an organism that can intervene with agency in the spontaneous evolution of reality—a reality that is neither static nor predetermined, but dynamic and in continuous evolution.

In the midst of this demanding philosophical quest, Needham had the good fortune of encountering ancient Chinese culture. In the heated debates on materialism and vitalism involving the entire scientific community in Cambridge, he in fact noted that, unlike everyone else, to his great surprise the visiting Chinese delegation of biochemists showed a remarkable indifference towards the whole subject. The new discoveries of quantum mechanics, the equation that brought together energy and matter, the dual nature of light (both particle and wave), and the idea of an ever-evolving reality, of which Man is an intrinsic part and never a neutral observer created no trouble or worries for these Chinese scientists. Consider that, in that period, the discoveries of the new physics formalised by Heisenberg, Einstein, and Bohr had literally wreaked havoc among the scientific community by forcing a rethink of the entire structure of Newtonian science. "This motion has caused the feeling that the ground would be cut from science," said Heisenberg; "It was as if the ground had been pulled out from under one, with no firm foundation to be seen anywhere," said Einstein; and "[it] has shaken the foundation on which the customary interpretation of observation was based," said Bohr (Capra, 2010, pp. 53–54).

Needham was to discover that Chinese thought could easily tolerate similar "revolutions" because it had never had to deal with the Galilean reference, but could, instead, count on a fascinating philosophical tradition which had never harnessed reality or reduced it to mathematical abstractions and fixed categories of interpretation.

The Chinese scholars he met at Cambridge were, thus, to have an extremely powerful influence on Needham. It seemed as if their stance towards the revolutionary new perspectives in physics embodied and offered him a freedom he had always sought. In discussing with them their traditions, history, language, and literature, he found something "equal yet contrary" to what he had been taught, something extremely deductive because of this. "But Chinese civilization has the overpowering beauty of the wholly other, and only the wholly other can inspire the deepest love and the profoundest desire to learn" (Needham, 1969, p. 176).

I believe the most interesting aspect of Needham's work is precisely this comparison he makes between two cultures that have evolved in different ways. Such a comparative approach in fact afforded Needham the heuristic means to discredit any idea of superiority or uniqueness of Western scientific thought and to historicise its birth through a critical consideration of its strengths as well as its limits.

The first difference, which might seem trivial, is geographical. The Mediterranean was a temperate sea surrounded by a multitude of peoples fascinated by navigation, which made possible commercial exchanges and early discoveries, with the merchant classes inevitably taking advantage. China was, in contrast, a large homogeneous area dedicated to agriculture where, after a period of fierce internal strife, a strong political organisation took control. The takeover was born out of a need for a central, unified power, which in turn could be supported by the flow of goods and tributes arriving from the countryside via an immense waterway system for irrigation. All this constituted the base for the regime of bureaucratic feudalism reigned over by the Mandarins—which lasted until 1912. The regime initially favoured the study of nature and its technological applications such as hydraulic engineering and associated mathematics, astronomy, the science of the calendar, medicine, and agriculture. Very soon, however, the rise of the Confucians and their ethos, which instated the supremacy of the intellectuals over the power of the military and over the creativity and wealth of the merchant class, came to block the birth of an equivalent to modern science. Thus, Chinese science never came to make use of either controlled experimentation or mathematics to verify hypotheses, the two pillars that, together, constituted the great methodological discovery of the Renaissance.

Nevertheless, this does not mean that China had no scientific development of its own. Indeed, as Needham states, between the third and sixteenth centuries AD, Asia was more efficient than Europe in the practical application of human knowledge to nature. This science was almost always state-sponsored, as opposed to the generally private character of science in Europe, and would be overtaken by the rapid development of modern Western science only after the Renaissance. Europe is actually in great debt to China for some scientific discoveries that, once imported, were to be key factors in our economic and cultural development. The best-known examples of these are gunpowder, the magnetic compass needle, and the art of printing. As opposed to Europe, however, none of the great discoveries made in

China ever managed to subvert, or were intended to subvert, the solid economic and social organisation of the country.

On the other hand, in the history of our own culture, the Renaissance, the Reformation, and the birth of capitalism are strongly correlated events. The merchant class was the driving force of scientific development because, as Needham rightly states, merchants were the first to move beyond the traditional separation between manual and intellectual labour. They understood the basic parity between hands and mind which was essential for the experimental method to take hold.

We owe Needham for his fascinating synthesis and original interpretation of ancient Chinese thought. His outlook is not the traditional one of a Sinologist or of a learned specialist, aloof in his absorption with his subject. Rather, his view is the result of the great curiosity and enthusiasm brought about by his encounter, as a Western scientist, with the appeal of a philosophical tradition other than his own. One which—in his view—managed what Western speculation had not: namely to fully express a view of reality which, while maintaining the rigour of scientific enquiry, by going beyond traditional forms could launch into an interpretation of reality aimed at maintaining all its complexity.

I find it intriguing that a great scientist, in the midst of his research, should have found in Chinese philosophical thought a mental attitude radically antithetical to that prevalent in the West: one based more on understanding than commanding, more on supporting rather than controlling, and, therefore, more capable of sensing and respecting the relationship between Man and nature.

It is no coincidence in this sense that Needham had a special place in his heart for the primitive Taoist school. He never considered this extremely interesting combination of philosophy, religion, proto-science, and magic, as a poetic form of mysticism; he rather intended it as a fascinating, properly philosophical, position: one that had a protoscientific aspect as well as containing a fully formed political vision in opposition to the Confucian order.

As well as asserting a well-grounded criticism of blind obedience to Confucian rules, Taoism in fact eloquently argued in favour of the need for a disinterested observation of nature as the necessary premise for its comprehension. However, their methodology never managed to go beyond empirical data because of a visceral antipathy and mistrust of abstract speculation. Taoists advocated that when the wise man deals with nature, he must be open to receiving whatever is offered, avoiding any preconceived interpretations. Chuang Tzu states, "Hold all things in your love, favouring and supporting none specially. This is called being without any local or partial regard; all things are equally esteemed; there is no long or short among them" (from *Chuang Tzu*, Chapter XVII, Needham, 1958, Vol. II, p. 48). The possibility of grasping the Tao is, therefore, strictly connected to the ability to rid the mind of all prejudice. "The mind should be an emptiness, ready to receive all things" (*Chuang Tzu*, Chapter IV, Needham, 1958, Vol. II, p. 48). "The sage is like heaven, he covers everything impartially; he is like earth, bearing up everything impartially" (*Kuang Tzu*, Chapter 37, Needham, 1958, Vol. II, p. 48). The frequent use of the symbol for water and the feminine in Taoist texts expresses the importance attributed to precisely this attitude of open, yielding receptivity in contrast to any sort of imposition. Taoists, in fact, defended all that is "feminine", the Yin—tolerant, lenient, flexible, mystic, and receptive—in opposition to the Confucian emphasis on the "masculine", the Yang—authoritarian, tough, dominating, aggressive, and rational. In nature as well as in human relations, an attitude of yielding and willingness, represented by the "Yin", was considered absolutely indispensable. "The sage follows after [things] and judges them" (*Kuang Tzu*, Chapter 55, Needham, 1958, Vol. II, p. 60). The ideal was to be able to "chariot the normality of the universe", refraining from any action contrary to nature. The *Tao Tê Ching* says, "Let there be no action (contrary to Nature), and there is nothing that will not be well regulated" (*Tao Tê Ching*, Chapter 3, Needham, 1958, Vol. II, p. 69).

The primal and general meaning of Taoist passivity was, therefore, to allow for things to develop in accordance with their own intrinsic principles, in order to be able to observe and grasp its *process*. In this empiricist matrix, resistant to abstraction, in defence of the scientific observation of nature, rests the principal influence held by Taoism in the development of Chinese science and technology, which, on this very premise, was thus more directed towards applied, rather than exact, science.

> To know that one does not know – that is high wisdom. The fault of those who make mistakes is that they think they know when they do not know . . . there are things which the eye cannot see, and which the understanding cannot apprehend, and which cannot be reckoned up in numbers. We do not know their how and their why. [Therefore] the Sage follows [Nature] in establishing social order, and does not invent

principles out of his own head. (*Lü Shih Chhun Chhiu*, Chapter 150, Needham, 1958, Vol. II, pp. 72–73)

The Taoist refusal to judge nature from an anthropocentric standpoint—defeating the temptation to make Man the only measure of reality and mixing his image into the surrounding universe—and its opposite recognition of the limits and relativity of human knowledge, translated into a deliberate disregard for not only abstraction, but also metaphysics, a tendency which came to characterise all later development in Chinese culture.

In its complexity, nature has always been a suitable field of study for the Chinese mind. For the Taoist, the Tao is simply the way the universe works, "the Order of Nature, which brought up all things into existence and governs their every action, not so much by force as by a kind of natural curvature in space and time" (Needham, 1958, Vol. II, p. 37). For this reason, the wise man must imitate the Tao, which works unseen and does not dominate. Understanding nature allows us to grasp the flow of energy and its organisation. Yielding to its order without imposing our own preconceptions is what according to the Taoists can actually grant us the possibility of taking advantage of it, "riding" its dynamics rather than engaging in a wistful and useless battle against them. Realising one's own nature, therefore, becomes the admonition of the wise man.

We find in Taoism a form of naturalist pantheism that underscores the oneness and spontaneity of the whole. The biological and inorganic are both governed by the workings of the Tao, which is present in every cosmic and biological phenomenon. "Returning is the (characteristic) movement of the Tao" (*Tao Tê Ching*, Chapter 40, Needham, 1958, Vol. II, p. 76; for the same concept see also Chapters 29 and 58 of the same work).

Even during the great neo-Confucian synthesis that occurred during the eleventh and twelfth centuries—when aspects of Confucian thought on knowledge and morals were mixed with the protoscientific attitudes of observation and respect for nature of Taoism—the keyword of the resulting new philosophy was *Li*. Literally "organised principle", Li however in no way implies the idea of a law imposed from the outside, but, rather, of a dynamic pattern operating continuously in all things, giving rise, at the human level, to social life and to the highest ethical values which can become expressed in it. According to Needham, the only Western term that comes close to expressing this idea is the word "organism". Therefore, in the Chinese tradition, universal harmony is not ordered by an instantaneous *Fiat* from some celestial legislator, but it is instead born from the spontaneous cooperation of beings following the intrinsic characteristics of their own natures. Here, in the idea of the spontaneous yielding of all things to their natural flow, we can see the re-emergence of the Taoist concept of *wu wei*, non-action (in the sense of non-intrusion): the rule of life that the wise man should adopt in harmony with what occurs in the world of nature (Needham, 1958, Vol. II, pp. 561–564).

The highest spiritual being known to, and worshipped in, ancient Chinese religion was therefore never a creating god, or in any case the depersonalisation of such a divinity occurred so early and so radically that it prevented the development of any concept of a celestial lawgiver committed to imposing his own order upon all non-human nature. Indeed, there is no word in Chinese to express the idea of creating something from nothing, so foreign is this concept in that culture. In their tradition the order of the world is intelligible not because it was imposed by a rational being on whose will the human ability to comprehend and express it would depend, but, rather, because rational human beings, the highest of all organisms, have been created by that same order and, therefore, have it embodied in their very minds. "Heaven, Earth and Man have the same *Li*" (*Chu Tzu Chhuan Shu*, Chapter 46, Needham, 1958, Vol. II, p. 581).

"Rational", moreover, in Chinese, does not mean intelligible in the Western scientific sense—in other words, reducible to laws which can be precisely and abstractedly formulated by Man. Indeed, the Taoist rejected, as we have seen, any abstract generalisation, but, on the contrary, postulated the relativity of human experience when dealing with the complexity and immensity of the universe. This, according to Needham, led them directly to an Einsteinian view of the world without ever passing through a Newtonian concept of nature. Moreover, as opposed to the Western stress on linearity, Chinese physics has always been ruled by the idea of wave.

> In a way, the whole idea of the Tao was the idea of a field of force. All things oriented themselves according to it, without having to be instructed to do so, and without the application of mechanical compulsion. (Needham, 1958, Vol. II, p. 293)

So, Chinese mathematics were always algebraic, never geometric. More than a logically coordinated symbolic system, maths was seen as a system of techniques capable of reproducing the concrete properties of the real world. The Chinese scholars always remained faithful to the use of the abacus and maths was applied to redesign the calendar; however, the methodology never required any strict proofing procedure, perhaps because formal logic never needed to develop as a formalised language due to the prevalence of correlative thought and the absence of the concept of law.

Chinese thought, in fact, never believed in the possibility of translating into strictly abstract terms either the rules of human cohabitation or the natural rules of physical order. Moral rules were simply a set of customs and habits—such as filial love or worshipping the dead—preached by magistrates, not to enforce but to persuade people to behave in ways that fostered their own and society's well-being. This kept the law much more correlated to the real and specific will and agreement of the people it tried to rule. This is far from the Western concept of natural moral law, which, instead, was seen as the expression of the will of a supreme personal god to be applied at all levels of justice and effective law.

In their language, and writing as well, the Chinese favoured the use of symbols that maintained an immediate connection with the real world; these symbols, in the connections and the resonance which unites them, aim to reflect the same network of interconnection, interdependence, and contextual influences that distinguishes the elements of reality they stand for. Concrete objects of reality were in fact never seen as isolated entities abstracted from the relationship connecting them with their surrounding environment and the continuous becoming of the whole.

The ideographic nature of the Chinese language well represents the need for a concrete language bound to an immediate representation of the object, itself anchored to a reality seen as a totality of things, actions, feelings, and relationships. While the Western mind asks: "What is this?", and searches for a presumed substance hidden behind the object, the Chinese mind, to understand one thing, wonders how it is connected—in its origins, functions, and purposes—to all the other things and how one should behave in dealing with it.

Needham believes the development of Western science was made easier by the very idea of a universal natural law and thereby the possibility for its precise, abstract formulation. From its inception, however, the Western idea of law is linked to that of a celestial legislator. "In order to believe in the rational intelligibility of Nature, the Western mind had to presuppose (or found it convenient to presuppose) the existence of a Supreme Being who, himself rational, had put it there" (Needham, 1958, Vol. II, p. 579). The natural laws that Kepler, Descartes, Boyle, and Newton thought they were revealing—notice how the term "reveal" is indicative of the assumption at the basis of Western thought—were in fact perceived as the blueprint of edicts promulgated by a rational figure that could be deciphered in the more modest, earthly language of rational beings through maths.

* * *

What has always fascinated me about Needham's thought is his invitation to reflect upon the origins of our certainties to object to the confident use we make of them. The journey into Chinese culture is only a way of escaping the predictable and allowing ourselves to be attracted by other possibilities. The aim of his critical comparison is not to establish which framework is better or worse, good or bad. His work is rather an invitation to reflect upon the qualities as well as the defects of the agonising culture we are part of: let us not forget that the twentieth century produced two world wars, the Holocaust, and Hiroshima. Needham suggests we let go of our intellectual hubris and find inspiration in other, different cultures that represent other ways mankind has reflected on itself and life. This is an invitation to a common effort, a philosophical effort, to improve ourselves by improving our understanding of ourselves and nature.

In the context of these reflections of mine, I wish to stress that, from the perspective of my own field of expertise, our culture's prevailing philosophical and scientific mindset has long made it practically impossible to focus and theorise on the emotional dimension of our existence. The organisation at the basis of our affectivity, in fact, has only very recently had the privilege of being becoming the object of scientific investigation. Furthermore, I believe that our implicit philosophical biases are the real reason we still have such difficulty being understood when we refer to the human being as a whole and, for a therapist like me, to the core importance of human relationships for the survival of the species. A detached, quantitative investigation has never been capable of understanding the organisation underlying the emotional aspects of entities as complex human beings, and hence they have been relegated to a vague, unscientific spirituality. Other cultures—although within their own limits—have looked upon Man differently. Allowing ourselves to "become corrupted" in this context means accepting what can help us adopt an attitude of reflection on the narrowness of our certainties and explore different approaches to reality, with the full knowledge that only other ways of thinking can lead to other ways of knowing and hence other ways of existence.

Given Needham's youthful restlessness towards the dogmatic structures imposed by the science of the time, so at odds with his natural tendency to perceive reality in a richer, more substantial way, it is no surprise, then, that he should have enthusiastically approached the Chinese worldview. In this culture, the human is immediately social, and this human–social dimension is not something extraneous to nature; rather, it is conceived of as spontaneously emerging from nature as a product of its eternal becoming. In the Chinese worldview, all things are linked by their resonance; there is no individual that, even in his individuality, does not participate in the life of the whole, where a spontaneous order emerges and reigns: an order not created or imposed from the outside, but one that mankind is agentically called upon to understand, respect, and reproduce at its own level of complexity, in harmony with the rest of nature.

Remaining confined within the Western philosophical approach, it would have been difficult for Needham to find a meaning-framework so simple and yet so very complex: a scientific outlook on reality disinclined to separate the parts of the whole. A philosophical worldview which, at the same time, carried within itself a strong ethical concern, one capable of grounding the painful questions that the twentieth century has forced us to confront with regard to our society—a West so apparently rich and powerful, yet so increasingly poor and fragile in its social relationships and expressions.

Critical views on Western science: Whitehead, Husserl, Marx, and Paci

With his organicism, Whitehead, whom Needham considered an ally, also started his philosophical enquiry from a critical reappraisal of a cultural heritage whose limits were already then becoming increasingly evident. And if the world described by philosophy has no correspondence with the one experienced in first person, the responsibility for this separation, in Whitehead's opinion too, must be sought in the past, in the historic development of Western thought. And, according to Whitehead as well, the decisive turning point—one that would become imprinted not only in philosophy, but also in the general attitude of all Westerners in dealing with the surrounding world and life itself—can be traced back to the birth of modern science.

How science was born—the role played by technological development in its affirmation, how the socio-economic conditions during the Renaissance impacted on it, the connections with the history of ideas in the Middle Ages, Ancient Greece or Jewish, Byzantine, and Arabic cultures—was then and is still a matter for study and debate. By investigating the ideological debt of scientific thought to European cultural traditions, Whitehead discovered in science—in spite of its apparent rebellious attitude towards the dogmatic and authoritarian rationality of the medieval world—the recurrence of a spiritual heritage still bearing the imprint of scholastic logic and theology. An underground permanence of the disavowed—not of content, but of structure—is often the risk in revolutions, both in history and personal life.

> Science thereby inherited the bias of thought to which it owes its origin. . . . What I mean is the impress on the European mind arising from the unquestioned faith of centuries. By this I mean the instinctive tone of thought and not a mere creed of words. (Whitehead, 1997, pp. 10, 12)

Medieval rationality had been replaced by another rationality, which, however, was *also* not free from absolute, metaphysical postulates.

Nonetheless, Whitehead's objective was not to cast doubt on the validity of scientific thought.

> If we confine ourselves to certain types of facts, abstracted from the complete circumstances in which they occur, the materialistic assumption expresses these facts to perfection. But . . . the narrow efficiency of the scheme was the very cause of its supreme methodological success. For it directed attention to just those groups of facts which, in the state of knowledge then existing, required investigation. (Whitehead, 1997, p. 17)

The success of this operation, when it was uncritically expanded to other sciences, Whitehead argues, has had a negative influence on the development of all European thought, as it was applied to domains where it could not work unless through a loss of complexity. Indeed, both philosophy and science took for granted an interpretation of reality based on a simplification founded on incomplete patterns of interpretation. With the passing of time, nevertheless, the immediate success of this viewpoint discouraged any attempt to verify or change its underlying assumptions. Therefore, Whitehead's position is not so much a revolt against rationality as it is a rebellion in the name of reason against dogmatic reasoning. "Thought is abstract; and the intolerant use of abstractions is the major vice of the intellect" (Whitehead, 1997, p. 18).

The "objective" world of science has entered our veins; and along with its triumphs, it has shown us an image of "the ultimate fact of an irreducible brute matter" (Whitehead, 1997, p. 35) in which elements appear as substances and/or qualities independent from each other, against a background of a space–time reduced to anonymous reference points, where phenomena are linked only by independent mechanical impulses. Western science has disconnected being from becoming, and irreparably separated the subject from the world of his experience, turning the cognitive-driven analytic outlook of the experimental method into the privileged link to reality, dismissing all other. By losing meanings in favour of so-called facts, the West has also turned the role of Man from the one of an active and responsible actor in the evolution of reality to a mere observer and consumer, presumed devoid of any ideality or project, even the one of looking after his own survival. It is important to note that even if science itself in its most recent evolution has had to overcome these dogmatic interpretational patterns, the "popular version of the mental state of the man of science" (Needham, 1931, p. 12), which still imbues our implicit ways of extracting meaning from reality in our everyday lives, struggles to shed an image upheld for so long.

If Whitehead coined a new philosophical language, if he used terms like "superject", event, "prehension" or process, it was to restore the image of a world moving beyond "scientific materialism". In opposition to it, he proposed a reality conceived as process, as becoming over time: a continuous passage from the potential to the actual, a universe where each event is related to every other event, to the entire surrounding world of the present, past, and future; this organised flow no longer something external or imposed from who knows where, but an integral part of the event itself. According to Whitehead too, then, the relation between subject and environment can never be an exclusively cognitive one—which would already presuppose a separation—but, rather, an experiential, embodied relationship: intuitive, aesthetic, emotional, practical, valuable, and meaningful. According to Whitehead, subjectivity, as it cannot be disregarded, must be restored, while the object needs to cease to be a mere "something" contemplated from the outside. How an entity becomes constitutes what that entity is; this is as valid for humanity as it is for the natural world: the two, although marked by a degree of autonomy, no longer separate. "Not only the life of humanity but the whole nature of the universe is processuality within space and time" (Paci, 1965, p. 131, translated for this edition).

The scope of philosophy, then, with Whitehead, becomes a critique of abstractions, with the purpose of restoring the profane, the immediate phenomenological experience, with the body re-dignified as a vehicle of sensations and activity and, therefore, information; in short, philosophy must recover the totality obscured by the selectivity intrinsic to reductionism.

"We are entering upon an age of reconstruction, in religion, in science and in political thought" (Whitehead, 1997, p. 34), and we cannot say loudly enough how urgent a rethink of our way of life is becoming: the negative consequences of the habit of considering life in a reductionist way lying in front of our eyes, every day more dramatic and severe. Consider, just to name one, the lethal effect that the idea of a mechanism with no values has had on industrial society, how "the doctrine of spirits as independent substances" has led "not merely to private worlds of experience, but also to private worlds of morals" (Whitehead, 1997, p. 196).

This, it may be argued, was the way the lack of consideration for beauty, both natural and artistic, characterising our contemporary society, was born. Beauty, in fact, from the new perspective advocated by Whitehead, is not just an aesthetic, surface category, but stems from a specific relationship between parts within a whole: an internal interdependence that Westerners have not been able to factorise and, therefore, safeguard as a value for survival. From this perspective, we can easily understand how it came about that we could blindly inflict such devastating damage to the natural environment, with the inconsiderate exploitation of resources going hand in hand with a trend of chaotic urbanisation mindless of the "relationship that connects every organism to its environment".

We can also explain how the excessive abstraction of knowledge has led to the development of professional specialisations that produce "minds in a groove", whereby "there is a development of particular abstractions . . . [so that] the whole is lost in one of its aspects" (Whitehead, 1997, pp. 197).

Scientific materialism has placed the accent on things and lost interest in values.

> This misplaced emphasis coalesced with the abstractions of political economy, which are in fact the abstractions in terms of which commercial affairs are carried on. Thus all thought concerned with social organization expressed itself in terms of material things and of capital. Ultimate values were excluded. They were politely bowed to, and then handed over to the clergy to be kept for Sundays . . . But the novel pace of progress requires a greater force of direction if disasters are to be avoided . . . we are left with no expansion of wisdom and with greater need of it. (Whitehead, 1997, pp. 197–198)

*   *   *

In the context of this line of grounded philosophical critique which has exposed the biases lying at the basis of Western thought, I believe that my own discipline, psychology, has a quite valuable contribution to make, and it can do this on the basis of its own field of expertise. Psychology, more than any other discipline, has in fact exposed and explained how human beings—far from being simple observers—are actors in the world of life, and how our actions and thoughts are not only moved by rationality, but also and especially by the power of emotions, particularly the ones which safeguard attachment relationships. Therefore, I believe that, with its contribution, psychology can enrich the concept of subjectivity, clarifying from a scientific point of view the emotional and environmental (therefore relational) requirements necessary for our species' survival. Emotions and attachments, in particular, appear to be the root of the sense of security that humans need in order to ensure physical and mental health. Psychology, thus, provides a rationale for their protection as non-negotiable values and for fostering their physiological development from the regime of infantile dependence to adult reciprocity, following the lead encrypted in our complex corporeality—which is never brute, inert matter, but, instead, always alive and biologically inspired in its emotional propensities.

*   *   *

Husserl, too, whose work I encountered through Paci, identified in Galileo and in the scientific revolution he started the change that was to "originally determine modern philosophy". This marked the beginning of a "positivism, [that would] in a manner of speaking, decapitate philosophy" (Husserl, 1970, pp. 42, 9) and create consequences felt to this day. All life before and outside science suddenly lost value. With different words, years later Laing would express the same concept:

> Out go sight, sound, taste, touch and smell and along with them have gone aesthetics and ethical sensibility, values, quality, form; all feelings, motives, intentions, soul, consciousness, spirit. Experience as such is cast out of the realm of scientific discourse. (Laing, 1982)

With the advent of Galileo's revolution, pure mathematics became universally applicable thanks to an unproved *a priori*: nature was reduced to a mathematical multiplicity, whose implicit corollary posits an universally exact causality. According to Husserl, through geometric and natural–scientific mathematics, we adapted a well-tailored, but *ideal* suit to the world of life. Certainly, by way of this, the West gained the possibility for a penetration into the workings of nature that infinitely surpasses the reach of a daily outlook. Husserl, however, warns us that we have taken for real what was only a method. One that has worked for centuries, for sure, but without any true comprehension of the real meaning of its workings and of the importance of what it left out. That is why Husserl calls Galileo "at once a discovering and a concealing genius" (Husserl, 1970, p. 52).

> Considering the world according to geometry . . . he abstracts subjects as persons . . . from everything that is in any sense spiritual, from all the cultural qualities things have acquired in human practice . . . world breaks, so to speak, into two worlds: nature and the psychic world. (Husserl, 1970, pp. 88–89)

The ensuing split between nature and spirit, between body and soul, has, therefore, remained *the* unresolved problem of European philosophy. It is, I believe, for this reason that the enigma of subjectivity has troubled the minds of Western thinkers for centuries. It could not but remain unsolved, because an explanation for subjectivity is sought only in vain through the method of the natural sciences. "Merely fact-minded sciences", says Husserl, "make merely fact-minded people"

(Husserl, 1970, p. 6). But there is an increasingly strong feeling of rebellion against a form of knowledge that, as a matter of principle, excludes the major problems of mankind, problems concerning the meaning, or lack thereof, of the whole of human existence.

We must, then, ask ourselves, "to what degree the exemplarity offered by science was legitimate and if those philosophical considerations to which we owe the new concept of the world and world science were not perhaps sufficient" (Husserl, 1970, p. 95)? Like Needham, for Husserl too, the transition from concrete to abstract is, therefore, legitimate, but only if it is conscious. Otherwise, the search for the right formulas might lead to the temptation to confuse the latter for the real essence of nature itself.

Husserl speaks of *epoché*, that is, "suspension of judgment", by which he means applying, in appraising reality, a wilful form of bracketing of our immediate conclusions, thereby gradually freeing ourselves from everything we have learned as obvious through our cultural heritage. In order to be able to perceive things that we have been blind to and discover a new, fresher way to see things, this operation must be conscious, in a perpetually renewed effort that is immediately translated into practical life. He advocates a rightful return to the ingenuity of life, the *Lebensvelt*, the world of sensitive empirical intuition, into which we are immediately immersed and from where every human operation begins, be it theoretical or not.

> In this world we are objects among objects in the sense of the life-world, namely, as being here and there, in the plain certainty of experience, before anything that is established scientifically, whether in physiology, psychology, or sociology. (Husserl, 1970, p. 106)

A world, thereby, in which we are objects among objects and, at the same time, the subjects who experience that same world we are part of: consider it, appraise it, and who refer to it through an activity conformed to purposes mediated by knowledge and culture. It is precisely the recovery of this immediacy of experience, of life giving itself to our senses every moment anew, of this immediate relation with objects and other subjects in the dimension of the present, in the legacy of the past, in the projection towards the future, that allows us to overcome the difficulties of objectivism and a mistaken subjectivism that continue to separate what was united in the beginning, bringing the overall awareness of the world to an "enormous enigma" (Husserl, 1970, p. 89).

Lebensvelt is, therefore, about claiming subjectivity back; in its immediacy, in the embodied experience of the world whereby the Self "intentionally" attends to the world of phenomena by continually and inherently giving it meaning, on whose basis, in turn, the Self informs his actions upon the world, thus constantly modifying the matter of his meaning-making, in a never-exhausted circularity.

We see here how, for Husserl too, reality is a constant becoming, whereby every man is called upon to participate in this becoming with his own intentionality and his own actions. Truth is no longer something established once and for all, no longer incarnated in an extraneous objective world to be contemplated from without by passive spectators. Truth cannot "be"; it "becomes" in a continuously renewed formation of meaning.

From this perspective, science, too, must be re-established or "refounded", meaning it must be recognised as a human activity endowed with its own validity, but itself in constant evolution, as shown, for example, in the recent turning point in physics regarding the traditional parameters of interpretation of reality. Returning science to its origins, in conclusion, simply means preventing its truth, or any other truth, from turning into an absolute, something fixed, which amounts to illegitimately extracting it from the flow of reality, thereby depriving us of the whole, of the complexity and richness of existence. Disavowing complexity, Man loses meaning, and meaninglessness renders the result of our own actions extraneous to our very self by making us forget the reason for which they were undertaken. In any case,

> when we are thrown into an alien social sphere, that of the Negroes in the Congo, Chinese peasants, etc., we discover that their truths, the facts that for them are fixed, generally verified or verifiable, are by no means the same as ours. (Husserl, 1970, pp. 136–137)

There is no objectivity that is not intentional and "the world already given has always become on the basis of human interests" (Husserl, 1954, p. 466, translated for this edition).

* * *

Therefore, in the minds of all these authors, the birth of modern science spurred the widespread diffusion of a specific mentality connected with the mechanistic, deterministic framework, which has increasingly concealed mankind's concrete and complex relations with reality.

History adds to our reflections by illuminating the precise link between the birth of modern science and the onset of a middle-class society. Based on this assumption, we might argue that, alongside technical and economic progress, bourgeois capitalism originated from and—more or less consciously—thereby endorsed an ideology that concealed the wholeness of reality. From a strictly philosophical point of view, it is, therefore, not a coincidence that the origins and foundations of Marxist thought, too, started off the premises of an appeal towards the restoration of the wholeness of Man. Here, again, we refer to the person in his or her concrete sensitive existence, whereby he or she is immediately active in relation to nature and other men. And it is precisely this restoration of Man in his immediate, sensitive, and concrete existence—before its meaning and substance is degraded by the interpretative categories of thought— that provides the philosophical foundations for Marx's criticism of political economy. Similarly, it is the realisation of the distortion lying at the basis of our idea of Man that prompts Marx's revealing analysis of Western science, which took him, too, to the conclusion that it has become a mental cage at the mercy of its own abstractions. This science, he argues, in the same way it illegitimately claims its processes and conclusions to be absolute, provides justification for the socio-economic system, classing it as natural instead of as the result of a precise historical becoming. Western science, according to Marx, hides and justifies under its apparent rationality the alienated relationships which our system has created between men and which we are no longer able to control.

It is no coincidence, either, that the field from which Marx's analysis drew its inspiration is political economy, whose core subject matter is Man's immediate relationship to nature. Analysing the historical evolution of how we have made sense of the rapport between subject and object in the specific ways the West has learnt to extrapolate meaning, we discover how, in our society, the ancient preference given to the "objective" disavowing the agentic and interactive nature of all human processes of understanding and meaning-making, has slowly led us to the total disappearance of the subject from our field of vision (Paci, 1970, pp. 388–464).

Even if concentrating on political economy and avoiding a more general study of the philosophical underpinnings of science, Marx clearly saw how the birth of science and the spreading of its mindset provided the facilitative environment and very rationale for the revolutionary transformation of medieval society into a capitalistic one. The spread of scientific discoveries, in fact, allowed for the development of new social classes that would eventually demolish the entire feudal hierarchical structure and, with the introduction of machines, gradually transform the old relationships of production. Furthermore, even though Marx recognised not only the merits but also the absolute necessity of science-based technology for Man to exercise any control over nature, he nevertheless attacked the way science has been, and is still, used in bourgeois society. Enslaved to capitalistic logic, technology for a long time now has in fact conspicuously not been aimed at fostering harmonious development or the satisfaction of social needs, but it has, rather, served to maintain established production relationships and pursue exploitation and profit for profit's sake, even at the cost of war and mass destruction.

* * *

In line with this trend of thought, Paci (1970) proposed that the crisis of science would actually be the crisis of the meaning of science for mankind:

> the crisis that Husserl discusses does not concern the sciences as such, but rather what they have meant and can mean for human existence. . . . Modern Man accepts being determined by "prosperity" and the success of sciences. He accepts, indeed wishes, to be a "mere *de facto* man", something that implies the reduction of "subjective" to factual . . . science is in crisis when, desiring to be reduced to factual science, "it disregards any subjectivity". To disregard the possibility for Man to shape the world is to disregard the "meaning" of human life. It is to believe that the "meaning of life" is either not a problem or that it is not a problem that can be dealt with rationally and, in a broader sense, scientifically. . . . Life, the psyche, and the spirit are not comprehensible as factual phenomena, as phenomena from which "specifically human questions" have been exiled. . . . Until now humanity has created philosophy yet remained outside philosophy. It has created science but reduced science to factuality, and would like to reduce Man to actuality. . . . The crisis of our age is the expression of that great phenomenon which is humanity's struggle for self-comprehension, for the mutation of itself and its meaning. This crisis requires a transformation which will be the more demanding the more radical the transformation which mankind must undergo will be. (Paci, 1970, pp. 19–22, translated for this edition)

The proposal of Paci—as well as that of phenomenology—to refound philosophy and rationality on new bases, letting go of the abstractions of positivistic science and restoring a vision of Man in all his complexity, implies re-assessing our views on our existence as human beings. This, in turn, calls for us to rework our understanding of the position of Man in nature by being open to perceiving and processing life in its pre-categorical, pre-scientific embodied essence and beyond the boundaries of the partial, simplified view afforded to it by modern science. Like the other thinkers so far introduced, Paci, too, locates the beginning of the modern era in the onset of the Galilean framework, by way of its false assumption that the mathematical idealisation of nature was, instead, a fact, a basic element of nature itself, and not an intentional act aimed at organising knowledge within an abstract system of reference. He believed the typical dualism of Western thought—mind *vs.* body—originated there, when Galileo's physical–mathematical science was taken up as the exclusive and unique model for all the sciences (Paci, 1970, pp. 26–50).

> The world of life is misunderstood and forgotten whenever it is concealed and hidden under the guise of abstract mathematical ideas separated from their origin, from real-life experience. . . . Abstraction has been projected onto life. Life itself has become dualistic. . . . The psychic sphere is differentiated from and opposed to the closed world of bodies. (Paci, 1970, pp. 35, 40, translated for this edition)

Against the dualism of Descartes, traditionally considered the founder of modern thought, Paci, along with Husserl, proposes the need to make a U-turn: a return to the integrity of the world of subjective experience with all its perceptions and emotions, and to its inter-subjective, relational nature. This would also imply a restoration of a sense of time as process, owning it through the recovery of the inherited, historical past, of the shared present, and of the future as that dimension of investment and project that gives meaning to life and, thanks to its ideality, creates an opening for repairing past inadequacies. No thought or feeling in fact exists that is not incarnated in a body "in the aesthetic concreteness of time". Life is the daily world in which we live; it is the "interrelation of people in first person". This psychological sphere, the field of emotions and intentions as fundamental constituents of human relational life which are strategic for the survival of the species, have, however, been left out of scientific theorisation (Paci, 1970, pp. 55–100).

In the mind of scientists, no suspicion holds that there "exists a third dimension: depth". However, the oversight of the embodied and relational nature of our experience is akin to a mental prison where scientists have self-constrained their worldview in two dimensions, losing sight of the fact that the factors they select as relevant are, instead, only "aspects of a three-dimensional world that holds a more profound truth". If the habit of abstraction and simplification has now become irremediably ingrained in each discipline, then "we must study not the field of one science separate from the others, but the acts of life, the operations of scientists in their own teleology". The new science, according to Paci, can and should be founded in the domain of the so-far-discounted "shared life", in the "world of direct, inter-subjective experience" (Paci, 1970, pp. 63–64, 70).

What I wish to stress here is how, through Husserl, Paci maintains the necessity to re-establish philosophy and all the sciences, starting from a reconsideration of their historical origins. He also shares the view that the basis of this revolution, aimed at re-introducing a long disavowed complexity shredded in the rush to find useful applications, can be found only in the return to a consideration of the emotional complexity of every individual who feels and of the inter-personal collectivity that acts upon and conditions that feeling. This, in fact, is the field that has so far either remained untouched by speculation or become the object of ineffective investigation using tools of interpretation strongly influenced by the reigning scientific model—still taken for granted, never analysed in their origins, never restructured on the basis of what the new discoveries have been trying to urge us to see.

This is somewhat similar to what happens in clinical work. Therapists are well aware that individual liberation from suffering passes through the reconstruction of what has been inherited and learnt from parental models, having the courage to overcome those aspects that turn out to be inadequate to guarantee survival and the full expression of individual creativity. Therefore, I believe that also in the development of history and culture it is legitimate, as well as necessary, to question what has been inherited and learnt as a given and taken for granted. This becomes particularly paramount whenever we find ourselves, as it is the case today, facing widespread suffering, a prevalence of injustice and tension, and a concerning rise of aggression, fear, and depression, as well as a collapse of economic and moral certainties. Obviously, such a dramatic state of crisis points out how the instruments used so far for the regulation and organisation of exchanges among human beings are no longer adequate, and new ones must be found. This task is necessary, yet difficult, since change involves a destabilisation we all fear, given our deeply rooted need for consistency. But awareness is fundamental to make this evolution a voluntary and well-guided course of action, and not just one passively endured. I think it is no coincidence that words like those of Needham, Whitehead, Husserl, and Paci, perhaps unknown to many, should ring so true so many years later, and should again become useful today, because those words were predictive of a development blinded by the very structure on which it has been based. Forty or fifty years later, we are in the depths of the crisis, but we should not despair I believe, as it is the very widespread and seemingly uncontainable suffering we are facing today that has the power, if we care to listen to it, to re-awaken us from the slumber of a progress only apparently free of faults, compelling us to reflect and look to science for explanations and remedies. I believe that science can still provide the very much needed guidance society requires at these dramatic times, but only if it first proves capable of analysing itself and owning its failings. That is, if science proves willing—as happened with the elaboration of quantum physics and relativity whereby scientists were forced by evidence to modify and correct their *a priori*—to reassess the certainties in which it has wrapped itself. These can be preserved for use in more restricted environments and areas, while science needs to prove itself humble enough to seek alternative and more adequate frameworks to apply to meaning-making in fields of investigation where rulers and numbers are not enough to keep up with the complexity of the events under scrutiny.

The revolution in physics and its philosophical implications

It might seem paradoxical, but it was the above cited discoveries of quantum physics and relativity that first forced the Western world to re-examine its own scientific certainties and reconsider their validity when applied to more extended and complex areas of enquiry than those in which they originated. That is to say, it was the very so-called exact sciences that first realised their own inaccuracy. If the Cartesian *cogito* actually led the West to identify Man with his rational mind and neglect our corporeity along with the priority that our sentient, embodied experience carries as the first agent of awareness, then

Newtonian physics provided a consistent mathematical theory of the world that remained the solid foundation of scientific thought well into the twentieth century. . . . The Newtonian universe was, indeed, one huge mechanical system, operating according to exact mathematical laws. . . . This picture of a perfect world-machine implied an external creator; a monarchical god who ruled the world from above by imposing his divine law on it. . . . When science made it more and more difficult to believe in such a god, the divine disappeared completely from the scientific world view, leaving behind the spiritual vacuum that has become characteristic of the mainstream of our culture. The philosophical basis of this secularization of nature was the Cartesian division between spirit and matter. (Capra, 1984, pp. 43–46)

All sciences were, therefore, modelled on Newtonian physics, and this model was to serve as a reference point even for those disciplines whose main focus is human nature and society. Biology, medicine, psychology, economics, and all the humanities, applying Cartesian reductionism, have studied Man and society as collections of elements that could be isolated from the context of life. After abandoning the model of popular medicine—clearly naïve yet more attentive to the organism and the environment—the clear division between body and soul led medical science to consider the body as a machine that could be acted upon from the outside to correct the malfunctioning of a specific apparatus. All environmental, social, and psychological aspects were completely set aside. Medicine ended up concentrating on the biological mechanisms on which sickness is based, attempting to combat them while neglecting any attention to the organism in its entirety and any role played by the surrounding environment.

In the field of economics, it has been argued that, before the Enlightenment, the long prevailing systems were value-in-use and barter, founded on the principle of reciprocity in exchanges. The idea of profit as we know it today did not exist, even in societies that already knew coins and money, and where taxes and salaries were in use. Only with the scientific revolution, the rise of the merchant class, the Protestant Reformation with its emphasis on the sanctifying value of work, and, finally, the Enlightenment, do we see the onset of an objective scientific approach to economic activity. This, too, was inspired by the prevailing scientific framework, namely the Newtonian idea of equilibrium and the laws of motion, on whose basis the system could thus be confident in a equitable subdivision of all goods through a theorised, spontaneous self-control of the market. We had to wait to the end of the nineteenth century for Marxist criticism to revolt against such a reductionist reading of political economy, raising how it buried under numbers and equations any focus on real, live human beings.

Towards the end of the nineteenth century, the Darwinian theory of evolution and Maxwell and Faraday's studies on force fields and electromagnetism also put the Newtonian model in doubt and showed the universe to be much more complex than Descartes had ever imagined; finally, with the discoveries of the new physics at the beginning of the twentieth century, a radical change was brought about in the concepts of time, space, matter, and around the nature of causal relationships; a change which would revolutionise scientific thought and create serious challenges for physicists.

> Every time they asked nature a question in an atomic experiment, nature answered with a paradox, and the more they tried to clarify the situation, the sharper the paradoxes became. In their struggle to grasp this new reality, scientists became painfully aware that their basic concepts, their language, and their whole way of thinking were inadequate to describe atomic phenomena. (Capra, 1984, p. 56)

From the point of view of materialism, it seemed impossible that something could be both particle and wave, depending on the point of view from which it was considered. Bohr spoke of "complementarity" as the heuristic making it possible to describe the same phenomenon from two different perspectives, as particle or wave, both necessary for understanding its complexity. He saw complementarity as a reflection of that inseparable duality intrinsic in how reality manifests itself which had been illegitimately split in classical thought, whereas only if kept together in dynamic tension it could be capable of restoring the idea of matter in movement. Matter as process could be made sense of by thinking of it as intrinsically equipped with a force, itself self-organising into different epiphenomena (*forms*) at various levels of complexity. "Thus the being of matter and its activity cannot be separated; they are but different aspects of the same space–time reality" (Capra, 1984, p. 71).

Since the discovery of the dual nature of light (and, shortly after, of the electron), matter, on a subatomic level, could no longer be seen as passive and inert, but was instead discovered as animated by a continuous motion, whereby stability appears only as the effect of a dynamic equilibrium. Therefore, mass came to be interpreted as no more than a form of energy and ceased to be associated with a substance.

Quantum physics also revealed how the world cannot be conceived as made up of isolated elements, separate and independent from one another. The inner workings of reality appear more like a complex fabric of relations in which the observer is an active part, as his presence contributes to the phenomena of which he comes to be an influential part, even just by being intent on measuring and describing them. Physics could, therefore, no longer be content with the illusion of a presumed neutrality of the observer, a neutrality that had been made possible only by pretending the subject were outside of the world he perceives. In sum, even in the physical world of apparently inert objects, there can be no objective observation. The only feasible option is participation, and, depending on the type of participation, different points of view and effects will inevitably emerge.

> My conscious decision about how to observe, say, an electron will determine the electron's properties to some extent. If I ask it a particle question, it will give me a particle answer; if I ask it a wave question, it will give me a wave answer. The electron does not have objective properties independent of my mind. In atomic physics the sharp Cartesian division between mind and matter, between the observer and the observed, can no longer be maintained. We can never speak about nature without, at the same time, speaking about ourselves. (Capra, 1984, p. 67)

If this is true for the physical world, we will see how this is even more important and inevitable in the world of affective relationships.

The role of the subjective frame of reference in the new physics is such that in the theory of relativity, even space and time have turned into mere modalities with which the observer measures and describes the natural world: not absolute dimensions, then, but themselves fruit of the observer's inherent egocentrism.

If we apply this to humanity and the development of science, this means that if we cannot disabuse ourselves of our anthropocentric sense, we should be reflexively aware of its relativity. Einstein's theory, moreover, not only powerfully reintroduced in science the concept of perspective, but also the one of environment. The contextual framework, in fact, becomes fundamental as an intervening factor for the explanation of events. Furthermore, forcing us to let go of the world of deterministic predictions, probability becomes the new tool for measuring what we *can* predict without losing sight of complexity. Probability, it might be useful to specify, is intended in this context as the *tendency* of a phenomenon or a state to manifest itself. Forced to let go of determinism, complex multi-factored causality, predictable in terms of potentials rather than facts, becomes the inevitable organising dynamic of a world not reducible to inert objects, but conceptualised as continuous becoming.

In sum, the worldview born out of the expansion of modern physics seems to irreparably lead toward an organicistic view of reality, in which all phenomena in the universe appear to be an integral part of an inseparable and harmoniously connected whole. While waiting for scientific authority to shed light on this new understanding of reality—along with the formulation of new, comprehensive, and adequate mathematical interpretations for it—for now we may still move around this new complex world by using the heuristic tools currently at our disposal, specifically complex systems theory. This, by way of a new interpretation of Darwinian evolutionary theory founded on a consideration of the body in its environment, has provided us with the scientific tools to explain the emergence of complex phenomena irreducible to the subordinate levels of organisation, but spontaneously arising from them. This includes the emergence of the mind and of human consciousness as awareness of the self and of the universe (Capra, 1984, pp. 239–240; also Morin, 1992, 2013). System theory, to some, may appropriately recall the laws of complexity–consciousness by the forgotten Teilhard de Chardin (Teilhard de Chardin, 1957, 2015), but also reminds us of the Oriental mystical tradition, which has always considered consciousness as the expression of nature's becoming and human rationality as a "living demonstration of cosmic intelligence": proof of the presence of a harmonious principle of self-regulation present in the entire universe, including Man.

*   *   *

In conclusion, in this chapter I have argued how a revolution in thought is becoming more and more necessary; a revolution specifically orientated towards re-balancing the relationship between rationality and emotionality, between mind and body, between adult and child. Only a different view of human beings and a reassessment of our real needs I believe can lead to a change that may allow us to escape from the decline that never before so dramatically threatens the survival of the species and life on our planet itself.

The current crisis, states Paci, is the result of the removal of Man and of his intentionality from our field of vision, in the name of a purely illusory "rationalisation" for objectivity's sake. This can be healed only by a return to our neglected subjectivity, to our affective corporeity, as Paci, quoting Marx, recalls: "Man cannot return to being a child, but should he not aspire, on a higher level, to reproducing the truth of a child?" (Paci, 1970, p. 357, translated for this edition).

The crisis now threatening the Western world affects the economy, preoccupied with production and growth and incapable of guaranteeing a more equitable distribution of wealth; the environment inevitably faces dangers, having to cope with a development indifferent to the devastating consequences of its energy consumption levels and of a model of growth unconcerned with the overall health of the planet; medicine and psychology find themselves confronting the illnesses of affluence and the growing existential unease that afflicts the world of the wealthy.

I believe that it could be very useful to understand that all of this is not occurring by chance; this is not the delayed effect of a necessary and inevitable historical process, but, rather, it is based on a conceptual error, a "misplaced abstraction" (Whitehead, 1967, 1997, 2010, actually spoke of "misplaced concreteness", referring to the violence of abstraction), namely a theory of Man and life barely capable of grasping the complexity that belongs to us, and incapable of making space for it. Along with the authors presented, I believe a reclamation of our embodied nature would be crucial to foster change, as it would point us towards the development and use of more sophisticated heuristic tools in order to gain a comprehension of reality that may not only finally give justice to complexity and interdependence, but also by that very measure restore the balance we have lost because of our indiscriminate use of undue simplification.

Basically, this is another aspect of the ecological debate, extended to include not only the threat to our physical health posed by the current disregard for the environment, but also a consideration of the impossibility of survival for humanity without a philosophical reclaiming of our embodied, emotional, relational nature and of the fundamental need to respect it. Ecology should, therefore, be expanded to include concerns regarding the mental health of individuals, currently damaged by environmental conditions unfit to meet our human needs. Ecology should also be concerned with denouncing the selfish, competitive, and aggressive mindset prevalent in our society and only erroneously attributed to "human nature". This in fact can be far more linearly and truthfully ascribed to the effects of the socio-cultural context we have created by denying our attachment needs. None of the predatory attitudes we witness in today's world in fact has actually anything to do with the healthy aggressiveness which nature has endowed us with to protect our existence—the idea of man as an opportunistic creature openly clashing with the interdependent, cooperative nature of living systems evolutionarily committed to survival.

The way forward seems to bid us, first of all, to take a pause and reflect. I believe change would be made easier in part by an openness to encounter the history of other men and other cultures, with the humility to integrate points of view different from those of a science that has reigned absolute for centuries. The aim is to restore integrity to what is complex and, with regard to Man and human nature, to integrate intuition and sensitivity, that syncretic parallel processing of appraisal that marks the domain of the "feminine". A viewpoint closer to corporeity and needs must hence be integrated into the mental attitude that has so far prevailed in history and science, one characterised by the dominance of the values ascribed to a distorted version of "the masculine", stretched instead well beyond its true and natural sensitivity and inclination. A reintegration of our logic with our sensitivity is the only standpoint whence it will be possible to build together a society and economy less adrenalin-driven and more endorphin-driven, less competitive and fairer, more capable of balancing the needs and interests of all, women and men, the latter restored to their original role of explorers of nature, inventors, as well as sensitive custodians of the natural family and of its survival.

After all: "within Man is a latent … humanity not yet born, but one that could be born if Man wishes, if Man takes upon himself the responsibility of becoming what he can become" (Paci, 1970, p. 22, translated for this edition), since "the meaning of truth toward which history leans is never completely fulfilled and requires infinite research, clarification and reconsideration, which all tend asymptotically toward the limit of truth" (Paci, 1970, p. 102, translated for this edition).

Note

1. The concept of emergence was developed within phylosophy and complex system theory and applied to biology, social studies and economics. We talk of emergent properties or configurations of a complex system when we observe, to quote Goldstein's (1999) original definition, "the arising of novel and coherent structures, patterns and properties during the process of self-organization in complex systems". A characteristic of emergent configurations is that "the whole is greater than the sum of the parts", meaning the new structure arising has properties its parts do not have and therefore cannot be reduced to the lower levels without a vital loss of information. The phenomena can be detected as operating in all realms of reality, from geophysics to biology to social sciences (Goldstein, 1999).

Mother, you had me
But I never had you . . .

Father, you left me
But I never left you . . .

Children, don't do
What I have done
I couldn't walk
And I tried to run . . .

(John Lennon)*

CHAPTER FOUR

A society based on a denial of attachment needs and all things emotional

It seems to me that the negative effects of a collective representation of life totally inadequate to account for the complexity of reality are for everybody to see. Fifty years on, my teacher's words still feel extraordinarily relevant and contemporary. With their nineteenth-century approach, the sciences appear completely helpless in facing the issues of a society in which technological development, because of the very effects of its triumph, is now called to deal with the dramatic issue of our survival, threatened by far from reassuring near-future scenarios.

If we observe the reality in which we live in the Western world—the so-called wealthy countries in the northern hemisphere—we quickly realise how the damages of a technocratic mentality coupled with frenetic development are becoming more and more visible and worrying. Despite this alarming evidence, however, our society is still held as a synonym of "civilisation", the one and only possible form of progress, and considered a model to be exported as if only the adoption of our economic system could guarantee the attainment of well-being and development. This attitude is so widely shared it is almost impossible to distinguish between opposing political factions, with only a slight difference of tone between Left and Right. Expert economists explain how the exportation of the neoliberal model, or globalisation, is instead absolutely essential, not for the poor, but for the rich countries to survive. Therefore, this indiscriminate exportation has taken place regardless of its benefit to the recipients, even at the cost of creating new victims in this senseless game: dividing previously homogeneous populations into privileged minorities and exploited masses, without the slightest worry about anything other than the immediate interest, or any concerns for the future we are creating for the generations that will come after us.

Yet, we are daily bombarded with distressing news. I am thinking, for instance, of the dramatic climate changes taking place globally as a consequence of human technological activity and the unrestrained emissions of CO_2. The effects of global warming are now self-evident, along with even more disastrous predictions of the near-future effects on land and sea as the increase in temperature and subsequent melting of glaciers and polar icecaps continues unbrindled. Effects like these are consequences of the wild exploitation of the natural resources so predictable that they could even have been predicted just by a good use of Galilean, mechanistic, deterministic science.

I am also thinking of the dangers from radioactivity, not so much as a consequence of war, though that is still dangerously possible, but as a result of peacetime activities such as the production of nuclear energy in the absence of a plausible solution to the problem of nuclear waste disposal. Naturally, this legacy will be for future generations, possessors of an imaginary future where we fantasise that there will be a science magically able to get humanity out of the corner into which it has painted itself.

I am thinking about an economy that distributes wealth and opportunities so unevenly that it divides the world into two halves, rich and poor, fuelling inequalities that inevitably spark dangerous social and global tensions.

I am thinking of the rhetoric about progress and growth that continues to promise an impending phantasmal liberation from living conditions that are, instead, becoming increasingly intolerable. This applies to both the Northern and the Southern half of the world, though for different reasons.

In sum, it seems that a "cognitive subversion" appears necessary if we want to finally dismantle the positivistic illusion that "scientific and technological progress necessarily and inevitably make living conditions better for the peoples of the Earth" (Latouche, 2004, p. 10, translated for this edition). Latouche recalls that the myth of our industrial age, born in Britain in the second half of the eighteenth century, brought with it the values emerging at the time in the Western world. Cut-throat competition, zero-sum thinking, limitless growth, and the unbridled plundering of natural resources became, therefore, synonyms of civilisation and progress, without the slightest analysis of the limits and negative consequences such a system might entail in the long course. "If all the inhabitants of the world consumed as much as the average American, the physical limits of the planet would be widely surpassed" says Latouche (2004, p. 41, translated for this edition). When he devised his socio-economic theory based on the need for a future "de-growth" as opposed to unbridled development, he also advocated "another kind of knowledge and another idea of science, one different from that blind and soulless, Promethean techno-science" (Latouche, 2004, p. 29, translated for this edition) left to us by Bacon and Locke; a science which, as I have argued in the previous chapter, is based on false assumptions. These have allowed for the justification of the sinister exploitation of nature to maximise Man's utility, under the false premise of a baseless trust in a natural harmonisation of the various interests, which instead came from the religious idea of a transcendent, omnipotent demiurge. We must "start to question the dominance of economy over life, both in theory and in practice, but especially in our heads" (Latouche, 2004, p. 42, translated for this edition), reintroducing "the social and the political into the economic exchange" and therefore "the objective of a common good and quality of life in social commerce" (Latouche, 2004, p. 28, translated for this edition).

Thus "de-growth" presupposes a criticism and challenge to those Western values which, for various reasons and circumstances, have prevailed so far over the course of the past few centuries. These have unduly obscured other values, regardless of their cruciality for our survival and even if present in our own culture, too. Only a retrieval of these human and social values may correct the dangerous processes currently under way. I am referring not only to the increasing threat to the natural environment, but also to the urgent need to intervene to re-establish a minimum of social justice, without which the entire global society seems destined to explode at some point in the near future. I feel we must therefore "decolonise the imaginary" and "de-economise our spirit" (Latouche, 2004, p. 50, translated for this edition) in order to save ourselves.

A bit of alienation

If we take a closer look, the current economic and social organisation— theoretically the best possible—compels people, even in the world of the rich, to live increasingly alienated lives. In fact, our lifestyle entails minimum, if any, respect for the basic conditions for human survival, or consideration for the quality of life itself, from both physical and emotional viewpoints. In parallel, we see an exponential increase in the rate of typical ailments linked to opulence: diabetes, seizures, and tumours on the one hand, behavioural and dietary disorders and depression on the other.

People are increasingly committed to extremely exhausting jobs, and by this I do not mean only the kind of work usually associated with fatigue, but also the occupations held as "safest and most comfortable". These are, in truth, becoming more and more gruelling because of the time demanded, the stress levels and the nightmarish performance levels required.

Indeed, work is considered life's fundamental—practically the only meaningful—occupation. It has lost its meaning as a means of providing for the basic necessities of life and expressing one's own creativity in that exchange of abilities and talents at the basis of our adult emotional world. Work is instead seen exclusively as a means to accumulate wealth, in turn taken as proof of self-worth. Young people are not led toward the careers they feel most attracted to, but instead they are urged into those professions which ensure the greatest earnings, in keeping with the idea that whoever earns more is worthier of social consideration, regardless of their moral profile. Public opinion is generally willing to turn a blind eye to someone who manages to accumulate riches even if behaving in ways far from the common interest. Money and success, even for someone who lacks both but aspires to having them, tend to push any concerns for the quality of our relational lives into the background.

The way our work is organised, under the insignia of absolute availability in the interest of productivity and under constant threat from ruthless competition, requires practically continuous performance and near total dedication in terms of time and focus: work hours easily take up the entire day, if not the night; sales points are always open, work shifts run continuously in both production and assistance, while only some of these shifts are actually necessary. This all-absorbing devotion to one's job takes time and energy away from periods of rest or relatedness, or, in other words, from those endorphin-inducing activities that—as is so wonderfully shown in the process of coming into the world—should alternate with adrenalin-producing efforts so as to guarantee the necessary balance for survival and for the full development of one's humanity.

Along with the idolisation of work, we witness how rest, vacations, and leisure activities, as well as relationships and emotional encounters, have been progressively emptied of their fundamental meaning and deprived of their value as vectors towards the full realisation of our psycho-emotional endowment. Instead, they have become insignificant corollaries, connoted by ideas of mere relaxation and escape, facets of life to which no commitment or effort can be dedicated, as resources are already widely squandered and exhausted at work. So it happens, paradoxically, that instead of dedicating the best part of ourselves to our most significant relationships in terms of our emotional health, we end up considering our home and family—far from the public eye and social scrutiny—as places where we can discharge the worst of ourselves; a place where we can be sloppy, tired, nervous, angry, or absent, with the absurd claim that those who are closest to us can or should more easily tolerate our estrangement, or, worse, our emotional excesses. Unfortunately, those who suffer the most are often our children, who have to put up with our inconsistent behaviours and availability (resulting from stress), since they have no option to defend themselves from their own need of us.

Even women, in their struggle to gain recognition of the value of their necessary contribution to a more sensitive and equitable society, have often bowed to the needs and customs of a culture marked by the dominance of a distorted, hypertrophic "masculine" (competitive, ruthless, utilitarian, opportunistic). Therefore, women, too, have ended up sharing a disregard for the importance of emotional values, conforming to the rush for riches and fame, while giving up any effort to defend an identity more attentive to specific "feminine" qualities. (I mean "feminine" and "masculine" as indicators of the basic, complementary templates and *not* as synonymous with "woman" and "man".)

Emotional absence within the family, therefore, applies to both parents, in the belief that natural requirements (in this case, the irreducible emotional and relational needs of the child, the meeting of which is a *condition* in order for him to become an adult) can be easily suppressed. It seems to me that we are currently making, in the field of attachment, the same error that took place 500 years ago when, ignoring its complexity and the consequent respect due, a scientific framework reduced nature to an inert object of useful transformation. Blinded then, as we are now, by the prospect of immediate gains, we neither reflect upon nor ask ourselves what could happen if the conditions for human beings' survival, in our inalienable physical–emotional integrity, continue to be ignored.

Even the school system seems to have given up on its formative role. Education is not intended any more as a fundamental actor facilitating development and, thereby, exercising a guiding and caring presence in extension of the family's role. One might wonder if schools are even aware of the responsibilities of their mentoring role in accompanying young people and starting them on the way to being better and more competent adults, which can happen in part, but not exclusively, through the transmission of notions. The education system nowadays appears to be intent on mostly stuffing young students with information, but it rarely *teaches*; it shapes professionals to fill the requests and expectations of society, but does not stimulate thought, or transmit culture, or think about forming reflective human beings and citizens. It is no surprise, therefore, if children and young people are increasingly adrift, considered only as potential buyers and, thus, subjected to a barrage of advertising and consumer conditioning. This is particularly serious as it takes place at a highly vulnerable age that makes it very easy for children and adolescents to take refuge in shared clichés, allowing themselves to be seduced by the models on television. They should be protected, but instead the latter increasingly acts as the contemporary babysitter of choice: free and always there, in the absence of parents and other adults truly interested in relating to youngsters and exercising their roles as carers and models of guidance. Thus, the young become easy prey to the most commercial and uneducational form of televised "entertainment", which transforms the poetry of life into a ridiculous mockery of sentiments, proposing a false promise of happiness tied to an idea of beauty untouched by time and to a success exacerbated by ruthless competition.

The contemporary "gods" of showbiz convey, to children and adults alike, false ideals, inciting consumerism while numbing minds and consciences. The social control exerted by the dissociation facilitated by excessive use of television and the new media therefore fulfils the goal of obliterating and suffocating any critical and rebellious outlook that young people and adolescents might bring to the adult universe. With regard to this, such manoeuvres in the service of controlling possible threats to the status quo are not bogus if we think of the evidence that the CIA, in the 1970s, had no qualms about distributing LSD—then a newly designed drug well known for its dangerous hallucinogenic properties—among young protesters who criticised the system and its stars. This was just another way to turn protest towards self-destruction. Today, drugs still circulate easily, acting to trap young people in a practice that quenches any aspiration for change, while, instead, encouraging mere escape from the squalor of a day-to-day life filled with too many consumer goods and devoid of any true values. Suffering and discontent are hardly ever investigated; instead, they are diverted and silenced by escapist practices that have the feel of a tragic surrender.

But even the god of work is beginning to lose its grip. The new *prêt-à-porter* framework of "flexibility" asks us—as progressive modern citizens—to be "elegantly" available to temporary and precarious employment, which instead impinges on the human hardwired need for security and consistency from the referents we depend on. Security, in fact, represents the foundation for being able to plan a life, dream a future, and even enjoy any sense of gratification from the recognition of one's abilities—human potentials which otherwise get lost. Precariousness, therefore, damages self-esteem, stripping contemporary adults—already deprived, if they have children, of any social validation of the cruciality of their parental role at home—even of the gratification stemming from their professional ability and commitment. Moreover, the current state of the job market sees those who enter the workforce, after years of exhausting studies with the hope of demonstrating and utilising their skills, often finding themselves with no work opportunities matching their qualifications. Young adults are, thereby, more and more often faced with the inevitability of adapting to humiliating work conditions just to get by, or else remain unemployed, postponing any plans for independence. From this perspective, it could be argued that the age of twenty-four established by the WHO as the general convention marking the attainment of adulthood is no longer adequate, while the number of eternal children–adolescents is growing out of proportion because of these external factors as well as a lack of proper facilitative environments fostering real emotional growth.

The economic and social organisation has created new urban and suburban landscapes. Urbanistic and architecture textbooks are full of any number of solutions capable of creating aesthetically acceptable and reasonably distributed syntheses between nature and culture. However, so far, these have, for the most part, remained only on paper, good for daydreaming; meanwhile, the spectacle of our cities and suburbs becomes more and more hideous. We witness the sprouting of clusters of housing built with no logic, dormitories added hastily to other dormitories, often the result of real estate speculations utterly unconcerned with any respect for the landscape or for the human need for a life as part of a social community. These new beehive-style domes, therefore, more often than not lack any plan for facilities such as schools, shops, and hospitals as well as transportation that would not force people into either isolation or private transport, consequently compounding to the congestion of our streets. This happens because these construction and building choices are solely based on the philosophy of business, profit, and, often, local authorities' corruption, and clearly not on a sincere desire for creating goods that are actually just that: human products aiming to improve the quality of life for everyone. And this pertains not only to under-privileged areas, such as we have in the south of Italy, where wild real estate speculations that have marred the beauty of the land can be too easily written off as circumstantial events, a regional problem generated by criminal organisations such as the Mafia and Camorra. The god of money and the logic of clientelism, instead, do appear to be the dominant values, everywhere. And it cannot be otherwise, until the role models celebrated by society and embodied in parenting posit a cunning and sly opportunism as the winning attitude.

In the end, even the worst things, once they are done . . . find their own rationale, their own justification just because they exist! They make those ugly houses, with aluminium window frames, unpainted balconies, unfinished block walls . . . people go and live there, they put up their curtains, put out their geraniums, hang the washing out to dry, get a television ... and after a while, everything is part of the landscape, it's there, it exists ... nobody remembers what it was like before. ... It doesn't take much to destroy beauty. ... So maybe more than politics, class struggle, conscience and all that other rubbish ... maybe they should remind people what beauty is ... Teach them how to recognise it. How to save it. ... Yeah, beauty. Beauty is important. Everything else comes from that. (Giordana, Fava, & Zappelli, 2001, p. 63, translated for this edition)

Privately owned automobiles, welcomed in the 1950s as a sign of widespread well-being and celebrated as the symbol of a new era of equality and liberty, have now transformed into one of the main causes of atmospheric pollution, even if not the only one, but still one of the main health hazards for those who live in the cities. In the wake of the partially mythical and certainly short-sighted success of the new technological era, many train and tramcar lines were eliminated, and with them any political focus on other means of transportation or on the introduction of limitations towards a reduction of emissions.

The glorification of speed, which has risen to a whole new level with the advent of real-time exchanges, means everyone is in a hurry to do everything right away, turning even long-distance air travel into an almost daily habit, where only jet-lag remains as proof of our uncomfortable but inescapable nature as fragile, embodied organisms.

Searching for a respite from increasingly shoddy realities and superhuman models of life, people throw themselves headlong into easy, consumeristic tourism. Masses of people seasonally travel to faraway places, less and less uncontaminated, searching for something that might remind them what nature and their relationship with nature was like before it was so blindly exploited and ruined, so that it can no longer be contemplated or enjoyed.

Big cities—inevitably I think of Milan, where I spent my childhood and grew into an adult—are less and less habitable, no longer places for stories and encounters, culture and transformation. Milan, for instance, but many other cities, too, has been reduced to a catwalk for the fashion industry and for a form of pseudo-culture celebrating an opulent and superficial modernity made of appearances, while the few remaining parks and green areas are fast-tracked to be soon sacrificed to "useful" skyscrapers and car parks. A perennial traffic jam grips the city in a stranglehold of noise, stink, and pollution, while no one seems to have the courage to oppose this destruction and defend a need for a basic quality of life. Cars rule in the city streets; pedestrians and cyclists, who evoke with their presence the possibility of a different rhythm of life and the pleasure of a casual encounter, constantly risk their lives, as is sadly shown only too clearly by accident statistics.

Forced to live crammed into spaces so far from being capable of meeting even the most basic needs for emotional survival, people seek refuge over the weekends and during holidays. In Italy, hordes of people routinely take their cars to move *en masse* to places of relaxation by the sea or in the mountains, where some hope of contact with nature is still possible. Places where some freedom from everything that makes us live constricted, programmed lives can finally be discovered, and another violated necessity can be restored: the pleasure of observation. In the same way, we witness an increased desire for cultural beauty, as visits to artistically meaningful locations are equally linked with the idea of escaping the city and an oppressive lifestyle. Naturally, the business machine—skilled in exploiting repressed needs for the sole purpose of profit—has extended its reach into leisure time through the tourism industry. By selling dreamy holiday packages, the system has created an antidote to the need for escape by taking advantage of it. All is well as long as no one complains or questions our way of life by investigating a little bit further the structural reasons behind such a powerful collective need to seek a beauty our everyday lives are so devoid of. So, people move in waves, resigned to traffic jams, long queues, and discomfort, while the healthy anger and aggression stemming from having to suffer this situation is redirected towards other victims; other people in line like you or travelling next to you no longer feel like fellow human beings with whom you might communicate, but mere obstacles and roadblocks along the way that spark hatred and competition.

People tend to adapt to these situations as if they were inevitable. I am always surprised, at public transport stops, when obvious and constant delays arise, that no one protests and everyone seems resigned to the situation. I have also witnessed, more than once, passengers express their indignation when they are told their train is delayed due to a recent suicide on the tracks. The bitter comments usually take it out on the disturbing method chosen by the victim to carry out this tragic act: "With all the ways at hand to kill yourself!"— as though the victim wilfully and shamelessly chose to interfere with the schedules of other people on purpose. How dare someone's human emotion of despair delay and hinder others from their hectic efficiency? How selfish.

This also reminds me of the uproar I caused some time ago in the apartment building into which I had recently moved when I innocently decided to put some geraniums on the windowsill of my mezzanine flat. My ingenuous purpose was to beautify and brighten up the façade, and the street, to everyone's advantage. I found myself instead served by the local police with an order instructing me to remove the flowers, as a result of some of my neighbours' formal complaints. Naturally, I did not give in so easily, and my flowers continue to brighten my windows. In the absence of any law forbidding me to exhibit these flowers, I still wondered how my gesture could irritate anyone to such an extent. I only understood when this incident was followed by protests against the colour I had chosen for my shutters—"too yellow"—and by the scandal I caused by parking within the appropriate lines and not invading the sidewalk like everyone else did. My neighbours' discomfort with me, I reflected, must be related to the fact that I had unintentionally shown a model of life that was "too liberated" compared to the resigned, grey habits of the other people living in my tower block. I came to the conclusion that my originality, suggesting a discreet yet rebellious fantasy in contrast to the reigning dullness, must have triggered anxiety and rejection because it suggested the scary prospect that small change *could* be within everyone's reach; a change, however, threatening the status quo, as it implied a possible transformation of the values on which our lifestyle is based; a change that anyone could benefit from and contribute to, if only at the cost of having the courage to put our certainties under scrutiny.

In a setting organised like our contemporary cities, those who suffer the most are old people and children: not surprisingly, those who are "non-productive" because they are either no longer or not yet producing. Municipalities, aligned with an idea of urban spaces designed and organised for active, wealth-creating adults, conspicuously never spend time or effort introducing spaces or paying attention to the needs of those who are carriers of another type of values, not easily monetised. In Milan, some years ago, someone had the bright idea of protecting the elderly from the scorching summer heat—in a city that is trapped in the suffocating grip of concrete—by parking them in the freezer sections of supermarkets—those areas, just to be clear, where I have to wear a padded jersey to keep me warm while shopping to save myself from the blasting air conditioning. One elderly citizen, in fact, caught pneumonia and died. And yet, it routinely takes committees and protest marches to protect the last remaining small greens and squares where a few old trees still cast a bit of cool shade on a couple of benches.

Children, led by the hand or pushed in a stroller, breathe their daily dose of carbon dioxide and noxious fumes directly from the source, since they are just about level with the surrounding cars' exhaust pipes. The less fortunate children are packed up and sent off to nurseries, undergoing precocious separations that are never recognised as such, but instead disguised and passed off as a chance to foster socialising among peers. This when, neurologically, a baby is still at a phase when no peer relatedness can be physically possible or enjoyable. The limited play areas are seldom protected from traffic and litter. I remember one of my children, when I took her to play in a rare green space equipped with a slide near my house, diligently collecting the cigarette butts she found scattered in the grass, examining each one in wonder as if it were part of the natural landscape. At that point, I decided there was no choice but to protect my children's imagination by escaping to suburbia in search of a hint of meadows and flowers.

With its inhuman pace, work has come to rule our very existence, even in terms of self-esteem, becoming the most important objective of adult life: something to which we dedicate the maximum of our vitality and practically all our developmental energy growing up, by channelling it into our schooling. We seem to think that the rest of our abilities and growth, including emotional growth, can be acquired automatically, with no special effort or dedication, as if nature alone provided for making the individual mature with the passing of time. And yet, just as we would die without feeding or caring for ourselves, so the need is just as crucial for a human being to be surrounded by an adequate environment in order to grow not only physically, but also emotionally and mentally. Instead, we take it for granted that children should adapt to their parents' absence without bothering to consider the time and consistent quality of availability needed to internalise the security and safety of a paternal and maternal presence. We fail to ask what a young mind's experience of being alive entails, or what children really need in order to grow. More recently, as new trends in child-rearing practices become more widely known, we trick ourselves by applying the idea that quality can make up for quantity and consistency of time spent together. This can, indeed, apply to later stages, but I'm afraid nothing can make up for the presence and experience of attuned relationships in the early years. These are biological requirements, in fact, when the building of the basic security that makes up the background to that slow and gradual path to emancipation from dependence must take place, lest emotional growth is stunned. We easily and unwittingly renounce the pleasures of parenthood, an extraordinary biological task that allows us to transmit our own life experiences beyond ourselves. Limited time, on the contrary, blocks that deep participation and dedication irreducibly needed for the baby to grow and for the older child to cope. Politically incorrect as it may be, science tells us that it is simply not enough to ensure the superficial presence of parents in the evenings, when they are already exhausted and worn out by work requirements and commitments. In this way, in fact, carers are forced to reserve for their children not the best of themselves, but the leftovers of an energy already mostly consumed. In this scenario, it is only normal that children's needs are experienced as yet another burden or duty for the adult to cope with. All pleasure is gone, and with it the gist of what needs to pass. It is impossible to fool ourselves into thinking that children do not feel this, although all they can do is try to adapt, beginning to doubt being truly important and loved, since they have no other justification to explain to themselves such painful absences and the look of snappy exhaustion of the parent when at home. Even though this applies to mothers first and foremost, as it hinders the fulfilment of that primordial need of a human child to feel confirmed and accepted by a mother's love—a requirement for the child's growth—it also dramatically affects fathers, rarely capable of dedicating time and passion to their role, one that is just as vital for the growth of the child and the successful separation from mother.

The absence of suitable models creates a propensity for our children, once they become adults—at least by definition if not in terms of emotional maturity—to similarly neglect the fundamental nature of attachment needs in their own lives. The problem, therefore, remains and is passed on from one generation to the next, as evidenced by studies into the transgenerational transmission of insecure attachment.

The care of children and the elderly is increasingly handed over to others: nursery schools, day-care centres, carers, and grandparents. To quote Fritjof Capra, our culture has stripped certain "entropic" jobs of meaning and value, that is, those activities which have to do with domestic care and attachment; however, despite the fact that these jobs are not currently remunerated with money or social recognition, these remain fundamental provisions for the survival of the species. Without domestic, physical, and emotional care, human beings at the most fragile of life's stages, infancy and senility, cannot survive. But even in active stages of our lives, such as adulthood, the need for nourishment and for love remains a lifelong requirement and, if acknowledged, poetically marks the boundaries of the human domain.

> In our society, as in all industrial cultures, jobs that involve highly entropic work—housework, services, agriculture are given the lowest value and receive the lowest pay, although they are essential to our daily existence. These jobs are generally delegated to minority groups and to women. . . . This hierarchy of work is exactly opposite in spiritual traditions. . . . It seems that the high spiritual value accorded to entropic work in those traditions comes from a profound ecological awareness. Doing work that has to be done over and over again helps us recognize the natural cycles of growth and decay, of birth and death, and thus become aware of the dynamic order of the universe. (Capra, 1984, pp. 212; also see Latouche, 2004)

According to some anthropologists, evolution might have awarded women in our culture a longer lifespan so that they may perform the maternal role in place of their daughters, unavailable because of work activities outside the home. Nature would appear, then, to be selecting this substitute function in order to guarantee the survival of the species (Bertirotti & Larosa, 2005; Chiarelli, 2003). Nonetheless, I would rather that women re-appropriated their own motherhood and require society to pay the respect and consideration owed to this delicate task. I say this in part because the menopause proves that nature does not look favourably on this sort of hand-over. Of course, there are countries more attentive than others in guaranteeing and protecting women in their maternal role. Some Northern European countries, for example, strongly support women financially during the first year of motherhood (or even longer). This is a time when the mother's presence is fundamental to ensuring the child's gradual emancipation from symbiotic dependence, and some countries guarantee later a part-time work arrangement that safeguards the mothers' careers as well as facilitating a healthy gradient in the process of separation. In such a context, women are able to provide adequate emotional and educational presence for their offspring, without depriving either themselves or society of the fundamental female contribution to the management of social and political issues.

In any case, as I have said, fathers, too, should recognise the importance of entropic work with regard to the care and accompaniment of their children. The father's is also an irreplaceable role that requires time and attention. To say that all this is a luxury, that it is not possible, would mean thinking of our way of life as unchangeable, as if we were not the ones who created it, and, above all, that we consider it to be the one and only optimal solution to social organisation. Instead, we must remember it as having a specific historical origin, along with relative and possibly biased scientific and philosophical foundations; we must free ourselves from the "dead weight of economists" (Latouche, 2004, p. 40) and remember: "Development cannot be limited to mere economic growth. In order to be authentic, it must be complete: integral, that is, it has to promote the good of every man and of the whole man" (Paul VI, 1967, p. 2).

Ecological thinking should, therefore, be extended to counteract not only the harm done to the planet, but also the (just as dangerous for survival) equally severe damage caused to our psycho-emotional endowment. This, in fact, is under constant attack by a collective denial of the specificity of its requirements and the blind celebration of an a-critical adaptation to social demands. This instead quenches any recognition of our unique agentic potential, as human beings, which entails the possibility for us to create the context rather than necessarily submitting to it.

Change is, therefore, becoming increasingly necessary, not only "to avoid the definitive destruction of earth's environment, but also and above all to put an end to the psychic and moral misery of contemporary human beings" (Latouche, 2004, p. 50, translated for this edition). Turning this around would mean "rediscovering the real richness of expanding warm social bonds throughout a healthy world" (Latouche, 2004, p. 42, translated for this edition). A drastic reduction in work hours could be imagined that would allow us to also enjoy a contemplative dimension in life aside from production, making room for play and leisure activities. This necessarily implies a change in values, not in anti-progressive or anti-scientific terms, but, rather, actually using the meaningful contributions coming from sciences other than economics, such as anthropology, ethology, psychology, and neurobiology: sciences capable of fostering a more complete view of Man and a more comprehensive understanding of the conditions for our survival, mental as well as physical. Then we could stop discussing the rise in the GDP and re-evaluate the non-economic aspects of life, focusing on improving the quality of life for everyone, even at the cost of some self-denial and sacrifice, acceptable only within the perspective of a greater breath for our emotional needs. "We must decolonise our mentalities if we want to really change the world, unless we resign to the change in the world condemning us to live in pain" (Latouche, 2004, p. 50, translated for this edition).

The effects of the current economic and social organisation exert a heavy toll on the lives of everyone because, apparently, only human beings are capable of adapting to a custom that deprives them of the time and ways for nurturing the emotional bonds that are fundamental for their very existence. Furthermore, if we think about it, in our "affluent society", not even the material needs that belong to our species are truly met by the sedentary habits enforced by our current work and housing arrangements. For instance, ready-made meals consumed out of hurried necessity and compensated for by binges that are anything but healthy are becoming a social habit, rather than an alarming sign of an eating disorder. Noise, worry, and stress disturb our sleep and impinge on our minds and bodies' need for rest and refuelling. Habituation and resignation are widespread social moods. However, they cannot keep emotionality repressed forever, and, in fact, it eventually bursts out, crying for justice, slipping out unexpectedly wherever it can, attacking our health or sabotaging the course of people's lives, heading them off the set track, attempting to change them somehow, often destructively, to try to be heard.

I am sometimes led to think—with even greater discouragement than Whitehead, who in his time could at least still witness a vestige of celebration of values, even if only at Sunday mass—that in this "reductionism" of life, which considers feelings superfluous, the privileged space for expressing passions has become sports: in Italy and in the UK, football, where rooting for one's team appears to summarise and concentrate love, hate, hope, dejection, joy, and anger, easily reaching the dangerous levels of violent fanaticism. I remember, in this regard, successfully helping a shy, lovely patient through the only domain where he could still get in touch with his emotionality in an otherwise grey life: his support for Inter, his favourite football team. He lavished on this team all the feelings he was otherwise unable to express in any other aspect of his existence. Even though he was a generally subdued, reserved person, the stands at the stadium were the only place he could truly "find himself" and vent all his repressed passion. The journey of redeeming his existence could start only from there.

*   *   *

The new media—some, like the telephone, television, and computer, present for over fifty years now—which started off as simple communication support systems, eventually transformed into virtual relationship partners and are increasingly replacing the chance and enjoyment of real encounters. Fewer and fewer people enjoy the printed page, for either pleasure or information, with its charms as a companion chosen and slowly enjoyed, with its embodied support's opportunity for annotation and conservation. People prefer zapping through quick, shallow, random messages, only apparently neutral, while, to add insult to injury, the flow of low quality, time-killing entertainment is obsessively interrupted by a bombardment of advertising to stimulate more consumption. Televisions and computers fill solitary evenings, giving the illusion of contact with the world, drowning the solitude and isolation of a society increasingly incapable of living and enjoying the pleasure of interpersonal relationships. Just consider the success of certain dating websites that promise the sort of romantic adventures denied by the reality of a way of life that forbids any space for emotionality. What is more, virtual reality creates the illusion of an ease and facility that does not belong to real life—actually even less so in our avoidant, relatedness-undermining society. In the task of construing real relationships, in fact, the limits of our physicality cannot be outplayed, along with the randomness, uncertainty, and effort we have to overcome to succeed, but this is also the only dimension where the possibility arises of the extraordinary charm of an accidental, unexpected encounter.

Objects meant to be useful become alienating and dangerous when they interfere with the complexities of our lives and needs, and when they divert, through unacceptable simplification, the needs of children and adults towards forms of gratification that are totally inadequate in addressing the real, underlying, emotional need. The widespread use of such surrogate ways of filling our free time remains unquestioned, accepted and tolerated, turned into a habit so widespread that it drowns any awareness of frustration. Any awareness of frustration would in fact be a threat, as it could turn into a collective, legitimate call for a way of life that could be healthier and more respectful of our nature. Technology, therefore, becomes somewhat of a dangerous mental drug, with effects comparable to those caused by the increasingly widespread use of narcotics in our society. Prescription drugs, often off-label, are in fact more and more frequently used by "normal" people: to get high and stop thinking, to overcome boredom, to adjust to the status quo, or to become artificially excited, escape oneself, or boost performance in order to measure up to the inhuman standards pushed by the psychotically competitive system our economy is based upon.

There is an ever-increasing dearth of adult figures who express a calm authority worthy of respect, what I previously described as "authoritativeness" as opposed to "authoritarianism". It is even harder—if not impossible—to find these among public figures: politicians, teachers, doctors, and experts from every field who should practise their professions with skill and selflessness (not in the sense of self-denial or martyrdom, but as opposed to narcissism), incarnating the proper balance of love for oneself and respect for others that should be the model for our offspring. The ignorance and devaluation of the emotional aspects of our existence has erased every trace of nurturing attitudes from our society. Such failure at modelling characterises not only its most obvious environment, the family, but also any area where the gist of a facilitating parenting template should serve as an inspiration and model. I am referring to any human relations where there is an asymmetry—teacher–student, doctor–patient, producer–customer—that implies listening, respect, and a performance aimed at satisfying a need to re-establish autonomy. Yet, as opposed to nurturing and facilitating, we see providing roles imbued with an attitude of mistrust, suspicion, and a preoccupation with defending the power of the authority, thereby maintaining the asymmetry.

Human relationships are objectified, seen as instrumental exchanges where the two possible roles are the ones of the retaining provider or the demanding costumer; the normal concerns of human relatedness are seen less and less in our interactions. Under pressure to follow excessively expanded and purely notion-based programmes, schools treat children and adolescents like inexhaustible containers of (often unprocessed) knowledge without allowing sufficient time for discussion, reflection, or the kind of assilimation that fosters truly qualitative leaps in growth. The concern is to create extended (yet superficial) skills. Little attention is given to stimulating the emotional process of learning that creates curiosity and reveals personal apti-tudes, which remain completely ignored and neglected. Anyway, it is the market that rules, not personal preference. It is becoming harder and harder, a luxury, to find employment in the area one really likes, for which one feels one has a talent. Like factories, schools churn out graduates for the satisfaction of a production system that goes its own way, following its own logic, which does not serve but uses minds and human beings for its own purposes. There is nothing more humanly offensive than to feel like a pawn, an easily replaceable object with no individuality, never gratified or spurred on by recognition of merit or the pleasure of feeling useful. It is increasingly difficult to go into studies and professions considered unfashionable or useless for the trend life in this society has taken, unless you are endowed with great strength and courage.

Our society's disregard for the phases of life—each in turn sacred—in its fleeting and inexorable course, and the collective denial of the unavoidable fragility of human existence, constantly disguised behind the celebration of a megalomaniacal omnipotence, makes everyone less prepared to live life as it is: in its beauty and frailty, in its need for a solid base of relationships to be faced, understood, and enjoyed. It appears that we have lost a deeper sense of our own exis-tence, one that can only be founded on the perception of an expansion of meaning proceeding from one generation to the next, each existence like the link in a running chain, where each and every one of us, with our own brushstrokes, contributes to a bigger picture and is called upon to add our own little piece in the greater tapestry of human evolution.

Instead, the cult we find in our society of efficiency and success, of youth and beauty at all costs, to be pursued by any means and with all sorts of aids—a message that children are bombarded with from an age that gets younger and younger—removes any meaning to the flow of life. We worship the myth of an eternal youth, untouched by time, celebrated for its appearance and superficiality. Sexual activity, made possible by biological maturation but not necessarily paired up with emotional growth, is mistaken for adult emotional expression and transformed into caricatures of public sentimentality and exposed bodies. Those who actually know love and understand sexuality easily spot these as cheap imitations, as they know the real ones must be a private matter, a gift exchanged in a secret reciprocity, for in intercourse we find the celebration of the invaluable emotion of meeting and a renewed surrender into trusted and welcoming arms. On the contrary, sweethearts are presently a pre-school phenomenon and parents are pleasantly indulgent. I dread the moment when this is anticipated in nurseries.

In our competitive and superficial society, relationships become yet another narcissistic battleground: I have (had) more than you; you have (had) less than I; whoever scores more wins. Don Giovanni, the melancholic antihero turned to model, is cheaply emulated. Love—or, rather, a mystified version passed off as such—is more and more something one buys: online, in special clubs, or on the street. Again, the illusion triumphs that money buys all: that one, having the financial means, can always compensate for a lack of real attachments—and, without them, for the lack of a sense of meaning in life. Through the purchase of an appearance, even fleeting, of love, we can delude ourselves that we can have what is missing, whose absence can thereby remain unacknowledged, as frustration remains disguised underneath the fantasy that the almighty power of money fixes everything. Moreover, in this "love for sale", we easily buy an apparent willingness that saves us the effort of looking for, and earning, through effort and commitment, the real thing; we avoid the disappointment and pain of failure and abandonment, without realising that, in such avoidance, we also lose the basis for any chance of a significant, fulfilling, emotional adventure. Indeed, to avoid the tedium of an endless repetition without real satisfaction, the realm of transgression is pursued more and more, in the naïve fantasy that shifting the goal of desire beyond all boundaries may finally satisfy rather than inflate its unfulfillment even more; this direction, needless to say, is the wrong one.

Schools for Yoga, Tai Chi, and Shiatsu are multiplying, and more and more people attend meditation classes and listen to the Dalai

Lama. These are clear signs of dissatisfaction with the Western materialistic framework and a search for alternatives to the dominant way of life. But with all due respect for the validity of these practices, they all seem like individual roads to salvation—pursued at times with absolutist fidelity, as if revealing the search for some missing saturation of meaning. Such individualistic pathways for escape are rarely transformed into the awareness of a need to change the system, to contaminate our West with a wisdom from other cultures; not because the West has nothing left to offer, but because it needs to look at itself from without to free itself from a blind and foolish intoxication with its own uninvestigated grandiosity which, in the constant celebration of our civilisation, prevents our society from stopping and changing gears as we face crisis. We are more and more urgently called to direct ourselves with new tools of awareness towards goals more compatible with human existence and survival.

The role and responsibility of psychology

Faced with all this, psychology—except for rare exceptions, and unlike in other, more glorious times in its history, when there was an air of renewal, and a more widespread courage in questioning conceptual norms—appears content with recording discomfort, when not actually contributing to its denial. Instead of using its voice to exert an influence on culture and clearly indicate the steps necessary for change and for correcting the system, it appears to be mainly concerned with inventing ever new and quicker ways to enforce mindless adaptation. Instead of siding with the irreducible needs underlying mental health, I'm afraid that psychology today, for the most part, sadly acts as a police force for monitoring and containing the crisis. In this, it joins forces with a mainstream, repressive psychiatric practice that, by definition and because of the instruments it uses, can only collaborate in maintaining, or even defending, the status quo. The use of prescription drugs, however useful and even necessary in the most serious cases, actually makes sense only as part of a rehabilitation programme that entails the analysis, comprehension, and removal of the causes of suffering. Yet, clinicians intent on finding the hidden causes and willing to expose the relational and social conditions responsible for mental distress seem to have all but disappeared. This, even though it is becoming more and more difficult to claim that these are simply private and individual illnesses, due only to genetic baggage or personal events, as we are faced with impressive numbers that would, instead, point to a collective origin to such widespread psychic suffering (Gerhardt, 2004). It is true that in mental illness it is the individual who suffers in his biological and emotional identity, in his personal history, in his hereditary and character components; however, it is our shared humanity which is offended, not only that of the person who becomes symptomatic. It is high time we recognised that we are all attacked by environmental and cultural conditions that go well beyond our histories as individuals, conditions which hinder or even prevent the natural, healthy development of our fundamental emotional nature as human beings.

Freud and the birth of psychology

Psychology has greatly evolved over the 150 years of its existence. Psychoanalytical thought, which first studied our emotional experience and recognised in it a depth uninterpretable by purely materialistic and mechanistic dynamics, has undergone numerous changes and developments since the first, primitive, Freudian model. Freud, like Wundt before him, started off with the ambition of founding psychology as an actual science, leading him to a-critically make use of the physics and physiology of the time as theoretical references. In the late nineteenth century, in fact, no other models were available. Therefore, in its beginnings, psychology used the prevailing scientific method as if this could simply be transposed to the study of human experience. All humanities, as a matter of fact, more or less a-critically transposed the model offered by the exact natural sciences on to their domain. In the study of subjective experience, the intuition linking psychological and biochemical processes was correct; nevertheless, this could not and should not have been translated into a reductionist approach. The resulting interpretational simplification, in fact, proves utterly unsuitable for representing human complexity. "For when science begins to treat man as an object of investigation, it somehow loses him as a person" (Guntrip, 1973, p. 16). However, even though the first version of Freudian psychology was strongly imbued with the impersonal conceptual mark of physiology, in the subsequent developments of its meta-psychology Freud actually straddled two different and, indeed, competing interpretations of human behaviour. In truth, Freud's biography and his own writings bear witness to the complexity of his character and genius (Jones, 1953; Steiner, 1973). Therefore, we must not be surprised that he was capable of oscillating, both theoretically and clinically, between an instinctual psychology and a personal psychology, somewhat going beyond—not without ambivalence—the prevailing scientific materialism of that period, which inevitably influenced and inspired him. He was well aware of the revolutionary character of his discoveries, but he might not have realised how they implied a radical rethink of Western scientific premises.

> Freud embarked on his psychological investigations with certain assumptions taken over from the natural science of his day, and learned from Helmholtz via Brücke and Meynert. These assumptions belong to the general outlook that is commonly called Scientific Materialism, and was the philosophy, or perhaps we ought to say the pseudo-philosophy, of most scientists at the turn of the century. . . . For Freud it was clearly as much a "faith" as any religious faith, which explains the tremendous emotional struggle he had to transcend the categories of neurophysiology in his psychological investigation. (Guntrip, 1973, pp. 121–122)

His own ambivalence notwithstanding, Freud's theory of the drives, the impersonal concept of libido and of the death instinct, the representation of constant conflict between impulse and reality, all show us how solidly the opposition remains in early psychoanalysis between the body and its needs and the mind and its rules, each committed to—according to Freud's perspective, inevitably given the theoretical means at his disposal—different, and even antithetical goals. In Freud's conceptualisation, we therefore find Man represented as traversed by an instinctive and impersonal current, the libido, imagined to respond to hydraulic rules. Before field theory, science did not have a model capable of describing needs as being rooted in corporeity in their physical and emotional components. In Freud's theory, the psyche is, instead, treated as an automatic mechanical machine that acts not for significant purposes, but to reduce tensions and maintain the quantity of excitement at a constant level. Thus, we see how Freudian theory remains constricted by the impersonal conceptual framework based on the physiology of the time. This conceptual stalling iterates the mind–body dualism and cancels out the personal dimension of the individual—as an organic intentional agent driven by needs and inspired by goals—in his psychophysical wholeness.

If I discuss the theoretical limits of Freudian thought and wish to underline the influence of the scientistic, deterministic framework of the late nineteenth century on Freudian meta-psychology, it is because, in my opinion, this is what has contributed to a loss and misrepresentation of its deeper meaning. Moreover, I consider it essential to preserve the awareness of how, even within Freud's original and central intuition of the importance of the emotional foundation for human existence, his inevitable alignment with the scientific concepts of the time involuntarily simplified the meaning of his own revolutionary perspective. This is why, I believe, the clear excitement present in the early discoveries of psychoanalysis was channelled into a scientific theorisation unfit to express it completely, thereby stalling their transformative potential with regard to Western scientific thought as a whole. I believe that in the same way physics passed from Newton to relativity and the uncertainty principle, so must psychology—possibly to an even greater extent—free itself from naïve mechanistic interpretations if it wishes to understand and explain the pressing existential malaise that increasingly pervades our existence.

Fortunately, psychoanalysis has moved beyond Freud, but I feel it is significant that Freud, in specialist or academic circles as well as common understanding, is and remains the most well-known and celebrated thinker in psychology. This a-critical celebration bears an influence that is extremely difficult to extinguish and which is responsible for that "popular version" of psychology that continues to feed, even in the layman, strong suspicions towards the impulses of the soul, considered hidden and mysterious, inaccessible, dangerous, antisocial, and, inevitably, maladaptive. Nowadays, everyone feels entitled to make jokes about slips of the tongue or lapses of memory; everyone throws easy interpretations, perhaps faced by righteous anger, be it a child's or adult's, resorting to "psychological" explanations involving *ad hoc* presumed envy, jealousies, or excesses and intemperance, allowing everyone to call everyone else who exhibits unwanted emotions "crazy". Most people feel authorised to pontificate and psychoanalysis, paradoxically created to uncover repressed emotions, has transformed into a means of, if not straightforward condemnation, at least suspicion and distancing from affectivity and its implications.

Freud himself, in the second topography, or version of his thought, which establishes the famous tripartition of the mind into id, ego, and superego, had to correct his original theory, complicating it with the recognition that the environment, through parental denials and prohibitions, heavily bears on moral orientation and a child's growth. He foresaw and discovered, partly reflecting on himself and partly through his clinical work, how much the educational atmosphere, imposed or mediated by culture, actually affects the emotional maturation of the individual and can be highly responsible for the development of pathology. However, not even in his second theoretical framework did Freud manage to conceptually overcome the core Helhmholtzian–Newtonian premises that defined and constricted the science of his time. The split between energy and structure remained, represented once again in the contrast between the id, on the one hand, and the ego and superego on the other, iterating the debt Freud owed to the inherited scientific ideology that continued to be dominant and unquestioned in his thought.

In Freudian theory, sexual and aggressive impulses consequently remain innate impersonal forces, indifferent to social needs and moral values, while the conscious part of an individual is thought to have to constantly defend itself from these drives, seen as inherently antisocial. Even civilisation would appear to have been born from this impervious battle by diverting the instincts towards other, "sublimated" goals; culture and social life would have no roots in the nature of the individual, but be solely founded on the repression of primary instincts. "On the face of it, it seems odd that our greatest achievements should arise out of the denial of our primary nature, and rest on our using for cultural purposes energies designed for different and anti-cultural uses" (Guntrip, 1973, p. 72). Instead, we could infer that Freud might have grasped the repressive, hypocritical character of the society he lived in and suffered from during his lifetime. However, he preferred to extol its qualities rather than emphasise its defects and limits—perhaps having little or no faith in his powers to change them. Not even the spiritual crisis that struck Western culture towards the end of the nineteenth century—masterfully represented in Freud's Vienna in literature and painting (Schnitzler, Schiele, Klimt, and Kokoshka) as well as music (Mahler and the young Schoenberg)—a crisis that, with all its unrest, doubts, and search for answers still did not manage to prevent Europe and the world from suffering two world wars in the twentieth century, nor succeeded to shake Freud from an understanding of the instincts as mechanical and hydraulic substances and bring him to realise the centrality of relationships.

On the contrary, because of his theoretical structure, which held him in a sort of insurmountable uncertainty, over time the unfolding of events only heightened Freud's personal pessimism. He stated,

> It is impossible to overlook the extent to which civilization is built upon a renunciation of instinct, how much it presupposes precisely the non-satisfaction (by suppression, repression or some other means?) of powerful instinct. This "cultural frustration" dominates the large field of social relationships between human beings. (Freud, 1930a, p. 45)

Freud, however appears to justify the oppression imposed onto the most natural tendencies of the individual on the basis that

> Men are not gentle creatures who want to be loved, and who at the most can defend themselves if they are attacked; they are, on the contrary, creatures among whose endowments is to be reckoned a powerful share of aggressiveness (. . .) Civilization has to use its utmost efforts in order to set limits to man's aggressive instincts and to hold the manifestations of them in check by psychical reaction-formations. (Freud, 1930a, pp. 58–59)

Freud's attitude appears as a wistful resignation, convinced, as he was, that the human being can be nothing but a slave to the blind, irrational forces presumed to constitute our nature and assumed as paradoxically acting against the Darwinian principle of the survival of the species. The doubt never seem to cross his mind that, as these unrestrained desires flared up in the dark, uncontainable aggressiveness which triggered the First World War and which he called the death instinct, the signs of a hidden, collective suffering could be found. That very suffering, if properly heard and understood, revealed instead the limits of an economic and social organisation full of hubris in its progress and science, yet unable to give itself balanced rules, and of protecting and fostering peaceful coexistence, because it was and is structurally deaf to the deepest needs of human beings. Freud shares with Hobbes, Pareto, and Schopenhauer a negative idea

of human nature, deemed as driven by forces of an antisocial character, which from his perspective could be held back only by fear,
through the sublimation of libidinal and aggressive instincts. He was
not capable of imagining that conditions could possibly be created
that would allow for a healthy emotional adaptation of the individual
within the collectivity that actually poses him in the first place.
Although incredibly perceptive, Freud's statements on this are pretty
disenchanted:

> We are never so defenceless against suffering as when we are in love.,
> never so helplessly unhappy as when we have lost our loved object or
> its love. But this does not dispose of the technique of living based on
> the value of love as a means to happiness. There is much more to be
> said about it. (Freud, 1930a, p. 29)

In sum, Freud senses what the problem is, but he had no means to
answer it. Freud's conception, therefore, leaves a lot to investigate and
comprehend, and I cannot disagree with Guntrip when he states:
"man has never hitherto understood enough of his own mental makeup to be in a position to bring about changes in himself in the direction of a more genuinely social capacity" (Guntrip, 1973, p. 71).

Fairbairn's turning point

In the roaring years of my youth, Fairbairn and Guntrip, Spitz,
Bowlby, and Winnicott, otherwise known as the British School of
Object Relations, were my fundamental points of reference to help
contain my frustration at dealing with the rigid Freudian–Kleinian
interpretations I was subjected to as a patient and which I had to study
as a trainee psychoanalyst; these interpretations seemed inadequate to
me also when, as a therapist, I worked in the last psychiatric hospitals
and then at the first Community Mental Health Centres. There, I
initially strove to make use of the principles of psychoanalysis in
settings that, with respect to the revered canon, left a lot to be desired,
or, better yet, a lot to be invented. Nevertheless, the passion was deep
and the challenge fascinating. Object-relations theory opened up new,
worthwhile perspectives for me in the understanding and healing of
psychic suffering.

The development of psychoanalytical thought after Freud saw the birth of various schools; without going into too much detail, I would generally describe some of these as created by dissenting disciples, while others, like Anna Freud's ego psychology or Kohut's self psychology, distanced themselves to a certain degree from rigid Freudian diktats or else focused their attention on overlooked details, in part because they were developed at different times and places. I have always considered these schools fundamental from a clinical point of view, because of their ability to suggest extremely stimulating ideas for treatment. In particular, I deem especially important for my own theoretical and clinical development those authors who shifted their focus from the analysis of adult patients to the one of children in their physiological growth. In the 1940s and 1950s, in fact, some theorists devoted themselves to the observation of children in their normative growth or studied the development of early symptoms due to deprivation of adequate emotional reference points, or, in other words, attachment figures. Among these, Fairbairn was probably the first and major author who completely opposed the Freudian hydraulic model of instincts with his theory of object relations, taking cue exactly from the unresolved and contradictory aspects already present in Freudian thought. Indeed, more than other authors, he provided a scientific–philosophical justification for his own beliefs.

Instead of dealing with erogenous zones and instinctive drives,

> Dr. Fairbairn starts at the centre of the personality, the ego, and depicts its strivings and difficulties in its *endeavour to reach an object where it may find support* ... All this constitutes a fresh approach in psycho-analysis. (Jones, 1994, pp. vi–vii)

Without questioning the fact that the nervous system acts with intrinsic modes of functioning, Fairbairn's understanding is that the agentic subject moves according to intentions, needs, and goals, which cannot be reduced to a mere discharge of tension. Excitement does not quiet down on its own. It is the encounter with an "object" (i.e., person, in psychoanalytic jargon) capable of an adequate response that allows for gratification and the ensuing relaxation.

> With Fairbairn psychoanalysis ceases to be a psychobiology of the organism with an ego-psychology tacked on, and becomes a psychodynamic theory of the person developing and fulfilling himself or being frustrated in his personal object-relationships. (Guntrip, 1973, p. 278)

What fascinates me about this crucial turning point is the realisation that the basis for understanding the individual and his emotional development lies in the relational element. This epiphany makes physical and emotional dependence a qualitative and emotional event, rather than a quantitative and physical one, as with the libido's dynamics; it further posits that only within this qualitative and relational event can we then individuate the basic biological foundation for the survival and very existence of the Self.

In Fairbairn, there is no separation between energy and structure, which was instead still implicit in the theory of the id, defined as the site of instinctive urges opposed to the ego as the site of control. Splitting and posing emotions and reason as conflictual, Freud had in fact implicitly and exactly reproduced in his metapsychology the Western conflictual dualism of mind *vs.* body and rationality *vs.* emotionality. "Freud's divorce of energy from structure must be regarded as a reflection of the general scientific background of the nineteenth century" (Fairbairn, 1994, p. 199).

> Had Freud been trained in the post-Einstein physics of the present day ... he could not have evolved a theory in which physic energy was conceived as an id separate and distinct from physic structure. (Guntrip, 1973, p. 148)

When Fairbairn and Guntrip wrote, and since the "Copernican revolution" in physics of the 1910s, in fact, the old dualism between matter and energy was slowly declining, as the dualism of light unearthed how they could no longer be conceived separate, but as aspects of a single reality to be considered in its entirety and intrinsic dynamism. As a consequence, over the course of the following decades, psychology, too, finally saw itself entitled to mould its theoretical framework to the new discoveries in physics, answering a general call upon sciences for a new respect for complexity. This turn might, in fact, have been what in the first place drove me to practise it.

Fairbairn, therefore, could propose a theory of dynamic structure in which instincts and impulses, no longer expressions of the impersonal action on the part of a hypothetical "libido", are seen as forms of energy and activity that express themselves in behaviours intrinsically endowed with meaning and directed at specific aims. This vision is prophetically in tune with the more contemporary biological approach that sees the organism as an evolving whole.

Fairbairn's thought entails a radical shift in the comprehension and interpretation of the aetiology of mental disorders, too; although this turn was made possible by the theoretical revolution in the framework of science led by the discoveries in physics, it was also encouraged and confirmed by clinical experience. It was, in fact, the latter that convinced Fairbairn that mental distress depended very little on a failure at controlling instincts, but was rather based on a desperate need for good object relations. "You're always talking about my wanting this and that desire satisfied; but what I really want is a father" (Fairbairn, 1994, p. 137) was the significant and enlightening response given by a patient of his that famously guided the psychoanalyst's reflection in this new, ground-breaking direction.

Going beyond the Freudian instinctual model, Fairbairn thus proceeded to propose and identify the passage from childhood dependence to the reciprocal exchange of adult love as the physiological pathway every individual, in his own psycho-physical oneness—an organic living structure, an energy organised at the specifically human level of complexity—has to accomplish in order to reach autonomy and psycho-biological maturity. Because of the complexity of the human mind and of the social as well as extended physical environment the human animal must face compared to other species, such a pathway is, however, much longer and more complicated than for other living species. The success or failure of this developmental pathway, moreover, is significantly dependent on the facilitative role played by suitable attachment figures; capable, that is, of nurturing and guiding.

In Fairbairn, the psycho-physical totality of the individual is present from the very beginning, already operative and experientially alive from the uterus. Although not fully developed yet, contemporary research has today confirmed that the foetus is able quite early to perceive the surrounding environment and to register its quality in terms of its capacity to respond to his needs. Overcoming the monadic instinct theory and replacing it with a theory of the *person* must inevitably include the role played by the environment as a cardinal element. It is the environment, in fact, that fosters, through its capacity to meet or thwart the organism's needs, a visceral and emotional experience of, respectively, either well-being or malaise. Going beyond Freud's idea of primary autism, Klein had already noted, through her own clinical work, the presence of an early ability of the infant's to perceive the mother, albeit in a fragmentary and partial way, at the first contact with her breast.

While staying faithful to drive theory, Klein also recognised the existence of a psychic life starting from birth, thereby implicitly shifting to an earlier phase the role and impact of cultural influence, with its habits and values, through its unavoidable shaping of the general attitude of maternal responsivity. Having absorbed Klein's position, Fairbairn, however, went beyond this, by firmly and explicitly ruling out the idea that psychological life was rooted on endopsychic factors independent of the environment and interpretable exclusively in terms of the antagonism between the instincts of life and death. Instead, he proposed that the individual's development of subjectivity could only be seen as the product of an *interaction* between environmental responses and an individual's genetic and biological endowment.

If Freud thought pleasure basically represented the experience of alleviating organic tension, Fairbairn turned the theoretical tables upside down, so to speak, in realising that the affective movement organising human behaviour is intrinsically aimed toward the object *itself*, not stand alone pleasure; in other words, pleasure can only coincide, physically and emotionally, with the gratifying presence. From this standpoint, he moves the theoretical focus from the organism to the person, from endo-psychophysical processes to interpersonal relationships.

If, for Fairbairn, normative emotional development is outlined as the passage from childhood dependency to adult reciprocity, and if, always according to his view, this journey is dependent on the presence of an involved, attentive, nurturing environment, psychopathological development could, therefore, be explained as an expression of specific types of partial failures in overcoming elements of childhood dependence; failures at coping, in fact, are bound to arise whenever a person who is only in appearance "grown up" finds himself confronting an adult task or role which he cannot possibly perform, never having moved beyond the affective structure of a child, be it overall or in that particular domain.

> Disturbed development results when the mother does not succeed in making the child feel she loves him for his own sake and as a person in his own right . . . the tone of voice, the kind of touch, the quality of attention and interest, the amount of notice, and the total emotional as well as physical adequacy of breast-feeding, are all expressions of the genuineness or otherwise of the mother's personal relationship to the infant . . . it is the breakdown of genuinely personal relations between the mother and the infant that is the basic cause of trouble. (Guntrip, 1973, p. 284)

As we have seen, all this acts against the perception of security needed by the newborn in order to grow.

So, the response given by the environment, in terms of welcoming, listening, nourishing, and caring, constitutes the first physical and emotional representation of the world for the child, and will directly bear on his trust towards life, which, consequently, will be registered as either trustworthy or hostile to his needs.

Central to this is the person, with all his or her emotional vicissitudes, and not only sexuality, which, although important, is only one of the emotional domains of adult emotional expression of attachment needs. "The cause of psycho-pathological developments would thus seem to be, not sexual or aggressive instincts, but 'fear and flight' from a bad-object world that the infant is too undeveloped to cope with" (Guntrip, 1973, p. 434). In this new version of childhood development, the Oedipal complex is, therefore, no longer the central allegory of psycho-neurosis. The Greek myth, in fact, offered a powerful embodied symbol of the notion of the irreducible conflict between "antisocial" primitive instincts and culture. According to Freud, the victory of the former would indicate the triumph of violence and lust—the antisocial drives allegedly intrinsic to the nature of human beings in his view—whereas a repressive culture would become the only means of survival for the species, with the unfortunate side-effect of making neurosis an inevitable by-product. For Freud, therefore, neurosis was a necessary evil, the lesser of evils. There would actually be a certain "recalcitrance of man's biological nature to the process of civilization" (Guntrip, 1973, p. 353). The only choice available to individuals, therefore, would be between giving in to destructive impulses or submitting to psychic suffering. From Freud's perspective, note that the environment is completely exonerated from all responsibility and, thus, it is not investigated, in the belief that any perceived environmental failure would only stem from normative perverse childhood imagination (again, alleged). In truth, Freud, in his genius, sensed the importance of the earliest phases of a child's dependence on the maternal figure, but he never developed a theoretical system capable of giving justification to its centrality and making it the basis from which it becomes possible to understand the trajectory of physiological development: that is, the pathway the little human being has to negotiate through the various phases of physical and emotional growth to become an emotionally healthy adult.

In Fairbairn, instead, an inextricable interplay between nature and nurture, genetic heritage and need for care, autonomy and dependence, is already present from the start, marked at every phase by a need for a specific balance of the two ingredients, initially proportionate to the small size and fragility of the baby. The slow, gradual transformation of this balance between these two irreducible human domains of needs marks the growth of the person. In this light, the oedipal struggle, if there is one, is only the sign of just one possible pattern of unresolved childhood dependence. In other words, the sign of a context-dependent uncertainty in the resolution of a specific stage of individuation which had made difficult, for that individual, the attainment of the necessary detachment from the maternal figure on his way to acquiring autonomy. The magical number three, so full of symbolism even outside psychoanalysis, and posited by Freud in his elaboration of the Oedipus complex as the key to a problematic epochal transition, returns in Fairbairn's vision of the natural family as the very guarantor of individuation. The slow, gradual detachment of the child from the original maternal symbiosis is, in fact, as we have seen, highly dependent on the fundamental symbolic and active contribution of the father figure. What was interpreted as the anxious adaptation to a castrating event—depriving and preventing the child from reaching the alleged happiness of an eternal relationship with mother—in Fairbairn and his disciple Guntrip is instead seen as the opportunity to apply the attuned presence of a healthy third party facilitating secure separation without incurring excessive anxiety. In Fairbairn's view, the father, from castrator, is, therefore, restored to the role of a supporting figure who accompanies the child in the actualisation of his potentialities; a figure who guides the child in the world, teaching him how to seek again the experience of that gratuitous, disinterested (as opposed to opportunistic) meeting which grants happiness in life, the first imprinting of which was already imprinted by the experience of maternal love. This is a meeting which, the father teaches, in the world of life goes from passive to active and is earned, through effort and passion, taking it upon oneself to reproduce it over and over in time, asymptotically.

Therefore, in physiological development, the third figure is the one who liberates, rather than the one who takes away, castrates or punishes. From Fairbairn's viewpoint, a punitive and castrating attitude would, therefore, be a sign of pathology, and not the norm.

Consequently, work must be done not to foster premature adaptation in children, and to make mothers and fathers aware of the importance of their roles as nurturing environment, meant to adapt first to the needs of the child and then effect disillusion gradually. Informed parents could then be able to commit to rebuilding, through their care, a place where, after birth, their child can find once again the safety felt in the womb, which, in turn, can accompany and support the child in exploring reality in a way that respects his ability and maturity.

The "good-enough mother" and the theory of attachment

More or less at the same time as Fairbairn, towards the end of the Second World War, other authors also came to the conclusion that the quality of the primary environment had a powerful influence on emotional development. With some differences that, unfortunately, I do not have the space to present in detail here, they all underlined both the importance and the responsibilities the environment has in the aetiology of mental distress. Further clinical studies, together with the observation of healthy as well as deprived or orphaned children during and after the Second World War, along with the development of ethological and neurobiological research and evolutionary psychology, all participated in bringing about a new awareness. In London, Winnicott was concerned with helping children who had been evacuated or orphaned during German raids. His observations had a profound impact on the development of psychoanalytical thought, especially in his underlining of the importance of a healthy relational presence for the psychological well-being of a child. Spitz and Bowlby also studied the tragic effects of emotional deprivation on childhood development. Spitz, aside from being the first to offer a description of physiological emotional development, movingly described the alarming "anaclitic depression" in abandoned children who let themselves wither away to solitary death in orphanages. Bowlby (1944), in the same years, observed at length and described the emotional reactions of children faced with an early loss of their primary attachment figures.

Although less interested than Fairbairn in theoretically justifying his position regarding certain aspects of Freudian thought, Winnicott—a paediatrician, great clinician, and insightful observer of the behaviour of those children who flocked to his practice for their health check-ups—focused on the centrality of childhood dependence and on the need for constant, adequate care for the full emotional growth of the person. He insisted on the initial relational unity between mother and child. "There's no such thing as a baby", he famously and provocatively stated, referring to the ignored but blatant fact that the neonate cannot exist as separate as he would be incapable of survival without his mother's care. We should speak instead, he argues, of a *nursing couple* which is still a complete whole, the same as during pregnancy. The experience of unison or unity is in fact fostered in the dyad by the mother's normative regression that reactivates her experience and "dialogues with" her own childhood experience of the world. According to Winnicott, it is from within this constant, ongoing relationship that, over time, the child comes to the discovery of the self as separate, through the slow integration of sensations that are both inseparably corporeal and emotional. The mother figure, recognisable through her consistent pattern of presence and modalities, is fundamental for this integrative work to happen. The new studies after the war therefore confirmed that Klein had been right in anticipating the mother–child relationship immediately after childbirth, but not in her interpretation of the child's seeking as exclusively run by the pull of instinctive drives. In the beginning, Winnicott observes, there is dependence and renewed bonding, long before any good and evil can be established. If the newborn searches for the mother figure with such emotional intensity (or "voracity", in Klein's words), it is only because the child has an *absolute* need for this: he must rediscover and re-experience the feeling of holding already felt in womb. The child needs this to re-establish continuity of his embryonic self-experience, since this is the only sensation he may recognise. This is an ultimate necessity for survival, Winnicott argues, not measurable by morals.

When confronted with the loss of their habitual context because of the war—such as their home, neighbourhood, friends, and acquaintances, an environment carrying an emotional as well as a physical value—Winnicott observed that mothers and children reacted differently depending on the quality of their attachment beforehand. He then began considering more specifically how the dyads already equipped with a solid emotional experience and, thus, "protected" by it, found it much easier to survive and adapt. These reflections led

Winnicott to his conceptualisation of the good-enough environmental provision (Phillips, 1988, p. 63), stating that a child needs a dependable, fostering environment, whereas the development of a death instinct would be nothing more than the physiologic reaction to an annihilating early failure of care.

> It seems as if an infant is really designed to be cared for from birth by his own mother. . . . [A] human being has to be taking the trouble all the time to bring the world to the baby in understandable form, and in a limited way, suitable to the baby's needs. For this reason a baby cannot exist alone, psychologically or physically, and really needs one person to care for him at first. (Winnicott, 2014, pp. 153–154)

Winnicott defines as a "good-enough mother" one who knows how to "initially deceive" in order to "disappoint gradually". Therefore, he considers the baby's needs to be so completely absolute at first as to require a response that reproduces as closely as possible the unconditional and absolutely contingent responsivity of the womb; only gradually will the child instead be able to cope with a demand for an active adaptation of his needs to the environment. On the other hand, Winnicott also described a pattern of responsivity that he defined as "impingement" which he discovered just as damaging as neglect. An impinging attitude is one incapable of *attuning*, that is, observing, listening, interpreting, and respecting the natural time-frames and particular ways of physical and emotional relatedness expressed by the child at any given time.

Attunement is so crucial for the newborn that nature provides the mother with a visceral preparedness to attune and adapt, through the hormonal changes that foster an identification with her offspring.

> [The mother] has, slowly, to disillusion the infant as to the perfection of his environment by mixing the meeting of his needs with 'graduated failures' of adaptation which do not go beyond the child's capacity to cope with and understand. (Guntrip, 1973, p. 401)

The procedure is made easier by the little one's natural growth and his own slow, gradual, and spontaneous evolution towards autonomy. Personally, I like to compare the good-enough maternal attitude with the rim of a blanket that slowly pulls back in order to let the child emerge with each newly acquired ability. Childbirth, in its intensity and gradualness, is, therefore, a powerful, embodied prototype of such a pattern of maternal emotional responsivity. The task of facilitating psychological birth is, after this imprinting, entrusted to the mother's own volition. She is called upon to be active after the passive role played in gestation, and a sensitive woman may be guided toward accomplishing this key task by imitating and completing the extraordinary model of physical birth. It is the way that other mammals, without the benefit of consciousness, know *how* to do. I can remember with affection and unchanged admiration the many kittens my cat produced in a box prepared especially for her on the floor of the closet. During the first days following the birth of her kittens, she had to be spoon-fed because she would not leave them alone even for a minute. As the days passed, she would allow herself brief absences that gradually became longer. During these, she would lie down at some length from the box, gradually increasing this distance and, thus, ideally outlining the area her kittens, now able to crawl, could securely explore.

> It is especially at the start that mothers are vitally important, and indeed it is a mother's job to protect her infant from complications that cannot yet be understood by the infant, and to go on steadily providing the simplified bit of the world which the infant, through her, comes to know. (Winnicott, 2014, p. 153)

This provides "not only the physical experience of instinctual satisfaction, but an emotional union, and the beginning of a belief in reality as something about which one can have illusions" (Winnicott, 2014, p. 163). For this illusion to hold in a child's mind, someone must commit to presenting the world to him in a way he can comprehend: in a sense pre-chewed, and offered to him in a "language" he can understand. In a certain way, with emotions and experiences, we should take a lesson from mothers in poorer countries who, without having baby food available, chew up little mouthfuls before passing on the food made assimilable to their babies.

To sum up, the big change brought about by Winnicott and, with him, by the British Object Relations school, who let themselves really read the suffering of deprived children during the Second World War, shifted the focus of psychology from a theory of sexual desire to a theory of the need for emotional nurturing, for being able to trust in the possibility of secure relatedness. Winnicott is one of those rare analysts who believe in physiology. He accused psychoanalysis and his colleagues of not having any faith in the natural human tendency towards development and growth. Psychoanalysis, being born not from the observation of a child's emotional life but from the analysis of adult patients' suffering, had committed the error of attributing to all children the fantasies and attitudes of those who had suffered from environmental neglect, turning them from a symptom to something normative.

As we have seen, neither Fairbairn nor Winnicott, even with some personal differences, read the intensity of a newborn's requests as the expression of a culpable innate aggression. Rather, they justified the infant's ruthlessness as an expression of the strength of the child's need for his mother in order to survive. Clinically, we know how the "all or nothing" attitude of our patients simply reproduces the perception of either holding or annihilation (as there is *no* middle ground for an infant) with which we are all initially confronted. Neglect is really and truly despairing for an infant, because a loving and caring presence represents, at this stage, *life itself,* whereas indifference or the absence of response *is* death.

"The theory that I am putting forward is that in the emotional development of every infant complicated processes are involved ... the completion of these processes forms the basis of mental health" (Winnicott, 2014, p. 159).

We must be grateful to Winnicott for having given us back a healthy image of the child, of his curiosity, his trust, his genuine, creative spontaneity, which should be respected and facilitated. A child should never be forced into renouncing his own naturalness just to satisfy the needs of the adults without whom he could not grow. According to Winnicott, premature adaptation to impinging environmental needs instead forces the child to build a "false self": a make-believe adapted identity aimed at preserving the attachment figure's goodwill, lest annihilation should take place. Winnicott observed, "Ordinary babies are not mad" (2014, p. 159). Possible symptoms are indicative of a suffering that requires interpretation. Moreover, all signs of malaise should be welcomed, as it is better if this is expressed, rather than left buried, leading to later, more severe, issues. This brings to mind another great Englishman, R. Laing, who, during the same period, faced with widespread childhood suffering, provocatively declared:

A child born today in the UK stands a ten times greater chance of being admitted to a mental hospital than to a university. . . . We are driving our children mad more effectively than we are genuinely educating them. Perhaps it is our very way of educating them that is driving them mad. (Laing, 1990, p. 87).

* * *

John Bowlby's work took inspiration from various studies on the effects of maternal deprivation in orphaned and hospitalised children; he built on the work of Spitz, Burlingham with Anna Freud, and later his own pupil, Ainsworth's, on the mother's role in providing a "secure base". Bowlby, similar in many ways to Winnicott but more eager to corroborate his conclusions with a theoretical justification, was the first to systematise all the findings of the early studies on the child's relationship-seeking nature in his "theory of attachment". He preferred to coin a new term rather than maintain the psychoanalytical definition of object relations, worried as he was about using a language capable of conveying the poetry of the mother–child relationship without penalising the concept of dependence. He in fact rightly feared that the term dependence would subconsciously evoke a somewhat culpable defect, when instead he was trying to refer not only to the extreme vulnerability of the little human being at birth, but to the life-long need for relatedness that marks our nature as human beings and which represents the very root of our strength, both individual and as a species. Even in adulthood, in fact, we need to attend places and entertain relationships that we can trust; Bowlby was the first to realise that, in our species, the need for a safe environment—for friendship and cooperation, for solidarity and empathy—goes "from the cradle to the grave". Moreover, he realised that intersubjectivity is biologically rooted as the only means of really soothing those feelings of solitude, danger and uncertainty that come with so many aspects of human life.

For Bowlby, this need for security that runs throughout our existence is, therefore, not only a psychological but a *biological* necessity connected to our intrinsic limitations; specifically, that all-human consciousness of our vulnerability—unique in this awareness compared to other animals. Therefore, attachment, he argued, has been selected as one of four psycho-behavioural innate motivational patterns selected by evolution to serve four fundamental needs for survival.

Aside from attachment, Bowlby named the need for nourishment, sexuality, and the drive to explore: all four equally non-negotiable, as the intense emotions that come with these activities provide an indicator of their nature as biological requirements. It could be argued that two of these psycho-behavioural systems—i.e., nourishment and attachment—represent the maternal and "feminine" branch of our interactional needs with the environment, and relate to the maintenance of our basic homeostasis, providing a psychological and visceral feeling of security; the other two, exploration and sexuality (in their underlying desire for otherness), oversee the need to separate from the family constellation—an internal drive towards the outside world which, as we have seen, is facilitated by the father figure.

Attachment is not a uniquely human necessity, but runs through the evolution of the species, serving the same needs but organised through, and distinguished by, species-specific types of behaviour. Moreover, Bowlby contended that the need for attachment cannot be reduced to, or enmeshed with, the need for nourishment. This was clearly evidenced by Tinbergen's ethological studies, Lorenz's experience with ducks, and, famously, Harlow's experiments with rhesus monkeys.

The little one has in fact an absolute need for relatedness, not just for food. Bowlby describes attachment—the profound, totalising relationship between mother and child at the beginning of life—as a biological necessity aimed at protecting the offspring from dangers and predators. He wonders, ironically, how the glaring obviousness of this evolutionary purpose could have been so neglected in modern, economically developed societies, where childhood behaviour had been studied taking for granted the wealth and comfort of the environment, while this hadn't been the case until very recent times. He advocated that this blindness had led modern theorists to oversee how not only physical survival (which can, indeed, be less threatened in the man-made environments in which we mostly dwell in the present era), but also the attainment of a basic subjective feeling of security for the child is biologically founded on his relationship with his mother. In order to be able to feed, in fact, one must exist, and we have seen how psychological birth cannot take place without the presence of a protective figure without whom the infant would not be able to cope with life and his own experience of being alive, even before we take into account the need to defend oneself from possible dangers.

According to Bowlby, the innate psycho-behavioural pattern facilitating attachment does not only organise the child's relatedness-seeking behaviour, but also complementarily superintends and innately prepares the parental response. Nature, thereby, would organise the instinctive emotional pattern of maternal and paternal affective holding in response to the child's cues. The way they will respond, however, is also heavily conditioned by culture, which can even overrule the parental hard-wired action-preparedness, intervening in the shaping of the actual expression of the response.

We see, once again, how nature and nurture pursue one another and complete each other; at the human level of complexity an interplay between innately prepared responses, conscious and subconscious processing—influenced by culture, values, and personal history—is needed in order to shape context-dependent, appropriate responses towards the common goal of enhancing survival. Survival, it should be noted, for human beings does not mean merely physical survival, but rather, psychological existence and the pursuit of the full actualisation of the emotional and creative potential carried by each individual.

> I regard it as useful to look upon parenting behaviour as one example of a limited class of biologically rooted types of behaviour of which attachment behaviour is another example, sexual behaviour another, and exploratory behaviour and eating behaviour yet others. Each of these types of behaviour contributes in its own specific way to the survival either of the individual or his offspring. It is indeed because each one serves so vital a function that each of these types of behaviour is in some degree pre-programmed. To leave it solely to the caprices of individual learning would be the height of biological folly. (Bowlby, 1988, p. 5)

Bowlby, as we have seen, reproached psychoanalysis for being blindly focused on the study of the adult patient without sufficiently considering the discoveries of developmental psychology or being able to utilise and be inspired by the insights coming from ethology; most of all, he woefully and insightfully noted how psychoanalysis had failed so far to play its very role as a speculative science and integrate the evidence coming from these more experimental disciplines into a strong framework which could explain and describe human psycho-emotional needs. In the same way, he argued, psychoanalysis had also been responsible for making any talk of "bad" families somewhat forbidden; even in the presence of blatant physical and emotional abuse, instead of recognising its causative role at the basis of anti-social behaviour and psychiatric pathologies among children, psycho-analysis had in fact maintained the Freudian diktat of unresolved infantile perversion as the only admitted aetiology.

> Healthy, happy, and self-reliant adolescents and young adults are the products of stable homes in which both parents give a great deal of time and attention to the children. . . . In most societies throughout the world these facts have been, and still are, taken for granted and the society organized accordingly. Paradoxically it has taken the world's richest societies to ignore these basic facts. Man and woman power devoted to the production of material goods counts a plus in all our economic indices. Man and woman power devoted to the production of happy, healthy, and self-reliant children in their own homes does not count at all. We have created a topsy-turvy world. (Bowlby, 1988, p. 2)

These, we may add, are the entropic activities and values that never enter into any calculation of the GDP.

Only recently, a growing number of voices have begun speaking out in favour of reassessing the fundamental impact of the actual caring provision given to infants. In a number of eloquently titled papers, Alice Miller, to name one of the most influential authors, has fully described the damages of an education that has historically been either violent and repressive or absent and indifferent, deaf to the needs and requests of the child. In *For Your Own Good: Hidden Cruelty in Child-rearing and the Roots of Violence* (2002), *Breaking Down the Wall of Silence: The Liberating Experience of Facing Painful Truth* (1997), *Banished Knowledge: Facing Childhood Injuries* (2012), and other papers, the author, with much courage and a stamina woefully rare to come across in this field, stigmatises how early neglect or violence—physical, of course, but also moral and psychological—have devastating effects on the growth of a person, making it nearly impossible to reach emotional maturity. Furthermore, Miller describes how victims of early abuse are often condemned to a mindless repetition of abuse of others as an ulti-mate, desperate, and useless defence against the memory of the trauma they suffered, as they have no other reference model for relat-edness but the one they have suffered and internalised during child-hood. It is important to stress how neither Bowlby nor Miller allude only to cases of explicit violence, although these are increasingly frequent in our news today, but refer more broadly to a widespread carelessness and ignorance towards the needs of the human infant—an ignorance which fosters and justifies improper, inadequate attitudes. These inappropriate templates of care—intrusive and/or neglecting— are often unintentional, but still harmful because they subvert the building of trust and, subsequently, hinder the ability for exploration and development. Without a secure base, in fact, one cannot grow and reach emotional maturity, but parents are completely misinformed as to the quality and meaning that should inform their caring provision. Bowlby sadly observed how our society's widespread ignorance concerning the nature of emotional needs promotes a chronic lack of adequate care, an alarming situation that no one seems to have any remedy for. What is worse is that people tend to habituate to the status quo, strengthening a false belief that nothing can be done differently and, therefore, things are fine the way they are.

Miller has applied her analysis to many famous figures in history, the arts, and politics to exemplify the repercussions of an inadequate education in their personal lives or, worse still, the effects of their psychic suffering on the lives of others, given the impact they had, through their roles, in society. It could be argued that her analyses might overly focus on psychoanalytical technicalities, and that they would benefit from being integrated within a broader historical, economic, and social perspective. Nonetheless, I think that the core of her criticism holds true, and that her writings still have a lot to offer. For instance, her historical reconstruction highlights how, in Western pedagogical thought, we find an ingrained, persistent, and deep mistrust of children in general. The little ones have, in fact, tradition-ally been seen rather like enemies—sly and full of boundless needs—a view that has provided a rationale for a parental discipline bent on keeping them under strict control; moreover, this negative view of children has historically justified the need to dominate their allegedly wild and defiant nature with a liberal use of cunning, trickery, lies, humiliation, and even violent punishment.

Although some of Miller's accounts from the "black pedagogy" might seem a little far-fetched today, they do resemble certain recent customs, unfortunately just as incapable of grasping and meeting the profound need for an impartial and sincere care which characterises human childhood. At present, manipulation and passive–aggressive psychological violence often appears hypocritically disguised as selfless availability, whenever the narcissistic needs of the adult are bestowed upon the child, thereby ignoring his real, separate needs. A regime of life centred around the needs and comfort of the adult, without the slightest respect for the times and rhythms of infancy, in fact constitutes a form of abuse which is just as damaging, as it violates the child's own developmental need for a holding environment tailored to *his* emotional capacities.

Another valuable aspect of Miller's analysis is that a study of the emotional deprivation suffered by famous historical figures and of how it impacted on their development and personality as adults may inform our reading of present-day figures. Just as Miller dealt with Hitler and Saddam Hussein, we are also faced with controversial figures in contemporary public life who, despite their dubious morality, have undeniably huge popular appeal.

In this regard, Miller's insights explain how generalised abuse and disregard for children's needs creates sympathy among the victims of similar abuses. If the recipient of this consensus is a politician, then we run the risk of delivering our society into the hands of those who act out a collectively-shared compensatory egoism, amassing their defences against the memory of the abuse they suffered by denying their need for attachment, and replacing the all-human quest for love with an unquenchable thirst for pleasure or power. The victims of abuse and neglect, in fact, having never achieved that minimum level of adult integration capable of fostering the advantages of correctness, justice, and fairness in terms of the survival of the species and quality of life, compensate with entitlement, greed, and resentment. Pleasure-seeking, power-seeking, and greedy accumulation of wealth are always the hollow mask of disavowed pain, anger, and fear: the long-lasting by-products of a chronic mistrust in the possibility of achieving full and healthy object relationships, probably never experienced.

The biological basis of affectivity

We have seen how the constrictions implicit to the Galilean–Newtonian framework which prevailed in Western science until the immediately past century prevented us from fully comprehending the complexity of the factors involved in the evolution and survival of our species.

As a consequence, until very recently, the world of attachment and emotions has remained foreign to scientific theorisation. The concept of nature has, for centuries, been simplified to brute physical matter driven by external forces, while everything that could explain inter-dependent dynamic processes has been considered a cumbersome surplus of little or no use.

> Although there had always been those who had known that the child was father to the man and that mother-love gave something indispensable to the growing infant, before Freud these age-old truths had never been the subjects of scientific inquiry; they were therefore readily brushed aside as unvalidated sentimentality. (Bowlby, 2012, pp. 7–8)

As the reader will have noticed, in this exposition I mainly cite authors from the years of my youth because I sometimes wonder whether the ground-breaking insights of the post-war period were actually ever read or applied, since they seem to have left little trace in the discouraging scenario in which we now live our "postmodern" Western lives. It seems as if they have been swept away, and it concerns me that this information and these thoughts never managed to reach the general public. Without any widespread diffusion, this important material cannot inform and create a fundamental social awareness of the real needs, rights, and duties that define us as human beings. The layman might still be surprised to hear that our survival depends not only on food—though this also is scarce in a large part of the planet—but also, and just as importantly because this is our nature, that we *require* a time and space for our feelings, for our emotions, and to cultivate attachments. Psychological knowledge has had little success in influencing medical institutions or schools, or in guiding economic planning, the organisation of work or of our urban spaces. Personally, I have never considered humanity's distinctive feature to lie in rationality, but, rather, in our varied and intense emotional richness. This because I observe and believe that plain ratio-nality alone, if not inspired and guided by emotional intelligence, can only move blindly and unwisely. Only feelings and emotions inte-grated with reason can reveal the flavour of reality. Without emotional information, our rationality would be useless and unable to orient and guide our actions. Alien to our Western tradition, the truth is that the two worlds of affectivity and rationality are not antagonistic, but complementary; what is more, rationality detached from emotion is a purely theoretical invention, lacking any neurophysiological basis.

> Emotions and feelings, along with the covert physiological machinery underlying them, assist us with the daunting task of predicting an uncertain future and planning our actions accordingly. .... Feelings, along with the emotions they come from, are not a luxury. They serve as internal guides, and they help us communicate to others signals that can also guide them. And feelings are neither intangible nor elusive. .... They are the result of a most curious physiological arrangement that has turned the brain into a body's captive audience. (Damasio, 2008, pp. 16–18)

Neuroscience tells us how feelings and emotions rely on specific biological substrata that make them possible and fuel them. The reliance on concrete, body-based mechanisms does not, however, compromise or diminish their informational and orientating value, Neither should their descent from an evolutionary process encompassing all biology impeach their status as an exquisitely human phenomenon; these bio-emotional roots, in fact, at the human level of complexity outline nothing less than what we have, for centuries, described as the soul. "Realizing that there are biological mechanisms behind the most sublime human behaviour does not imply a simplistic reduction to the nuts and bolts of neurobiology" (Damasio, 2008, p. 145). I do not feel that it is in the least reductionist to learn that adrenalin is at the basis of attachment-seeking behaviour, or that oxytocin and prolactin feed the affectionate exchanges of sexuality or the ones of the postnatal period, that endorphins accompany our pleasure and happiness, and that catecholamine governs defensive "fight or flight" operations, and so on (Schmid, 2005, pp. 44–54). I think it is fascinating to learn about the tripartite brain: reptilian, limbic, and cerebral cortex, which correspond, respectively, to the centres of cardiac and respiratory control, emotions, and cognitive and rational functioning. In considering this, we can see how the effect of a slow evolution functionally superimposed one on the other, revealing how there is just no physical possibility for content in the human mind not to be charged with emotional undertones, too. Any refined and abstract processing carried out in the cortex is, in fact, the codified result of content that first passed through the limbic area of the brain, or, in other words, processed in that middle strata where emotional and visceral data is collected as we experience life in the world

(Bertirotti & Larosa, 2005; Chiarelli, 1997, 2003; Gerhardt, 2004; MacLean, 1972). Rather than taking the poetry out of our mental life, I feel this confirms once again that nature has provided us with all the biological means, emotional and rational, to enjoy and preserve our existence.

Damasio states,

> The truth of the feeling . . . the magnitude of the feeling, and the beauty of the feeling, are not endangered by realizing that survival, brain, and proper education have a lot to do with the reasons why we experience such feelings. (Damasio, 2008, p. 146)

The above provided, of course, that education and culture are in tune with our human needs, starting from the child's, and never work against our nature. Neuroscience also informs us on how, even though it is true that hereditary factors play their part in the development of a child's character, it is his attachment relationships that will shape the architecture of his brain at the beginning of life. Gerhardt emphasises how the exchange of affectionate looks sparks biochemical reactions of pleasure, and how certain brain structures—the hippocampus, temporal cortex, and the rear and prefrontal cingulate cortexes—are not mature at birth but develop through the repetition of qualitatively positive experiences (Gerhardt, 2004, p. 50). "[The brain's] development must be seen . . . as the product of the effects of experience on the unfolding of genetic potential" (Siegel, 2012, p. 30). "In [early] transactions the primary caregiver is providing experiences which shape genetic potential by acting as psychobiological regulator (or disregulator) of hormones that directly influence gene transcription" (Schore, 1997, p. 616). "Each individual's history reflects an inseparable blend of how the environment, random events, gender and temperament all contribute to the creation of experiences in which adaptation and learning recursively shape the development of the mind" (Siegel, 2012, p. 31). It is, therefore, the relationship with caregivers that provides the first form of interpersonal communication, allowing the child's

> brain to develop a balanced capacity to regulate emotions, to feel connected to other people, to establish an autobiographical story, and to move out into the world with a sense of vitality. . . . These important early interpersonal are encoded within various forms of memory and shape the architecture of brain. (Siegel, 2012, pp. 34–35)

... at birth the newborn is faced with a range of possible paths, and the path he chooses will be determined at every step by the interaction of the individual, as he is at that moment, with the environment in which he happens to be. .... The particular path the infant will choose will be determined by the surrounding environment, especially the way his parents (or parental substitutes) treat him, and by how the infant responds to them. .... Since the course of subsequent development is not fixed, changes in the way a child is treated can shift his pathway in either a more favorable direction or a less favorable one. Although the capacity for developmental change diminishes with age, change continues throughout the life cycle so that changes for better or for worse are always possible. It is this continuing potential for change that means that at no time of life is a person invulnerable to every possible adversity and also that at no time of life is a person impermeable to favourable influence. (Bowlby, 1988, p. 136)

Indeed, even "as adults we [continue not only to] need to be understood and cared about, but [also] to have other individuals simultaneously experience a state of mind similar to our own" (Siegel, 2012, p. 35). Becoming an adult, in sum, implies the end of one-way dependence, but not of the need for emotional resonance.

* * *

I had the good fortune of meeting Franco Fornari (1921–1985)—influential Italian psychoanalyst and theoretician—and of working alongside him in the early 1980s in a training programme in the first Mental Health Community Centres. That was how I took part in his attempt to apply his method of "code analysis" within these institutions (Fornari, 1976, 1977, 1981; Pietropolli Charmet, 1987), and how I came to learn about his hypothesis of a biological foundation for "living codes". He intended these as hardwired affective "constellations" (not far from the ethological and Bowlbian notion of action-preparedness) which nature would have equipped us as emergent, potential "vocabularies" of felt experience favouring, in certain contexts, the activation of certain behaviours, appraisal modalities and attitudes associated with the survival of the species.

I found Fornari's idea very stimulating even though, because of my character and previous studies, I could only distance myself from his purely linguistic approach. I, in fact, personally found his reliance on language still too anchored to Freudian–Kleinian thought, so I eventually moved towards more markedly anthropological and biological research.

In these disciplines, however, I did find grounded, experimental support for his very theories, specifically for the existence of constituent hormonal and neuro-mental differences underlying paternal and maternal templates. These findings substantiate Fornari's thesis that these would indeed be innate and embodied complementary modalities of affective organisation, present in individuals of both genders—even though in different measures—which become activated in salient contexts. We can see then how evolution appears to have prepared for these "living codes", or qualities of appraisal and response, to come to be interwoven physically and emotionally in the care provision to increase the chance of survival of the child and the species.

In light of its visionary power and capacity to forerun more recent findings in neuro-psycho-endocrinology and neuroscience, I believe Fornari's theory still holds great suggestive power even though it can be somewhat arduous to approach, and I am going to outline it here for the reader's interest, convinced it may enrich this analysis.

Fornari maintained that human beings are pervaded with a "code of natural affective signification", which would function as an instinctive vocabulary dividing experience into building blocks of embodied meaning. These basic units, called "coinemes" would allow us to "familiarise and physicalise the world". He defined these units as "unconscious decision-making powers" that would give rise to basic affective orientations, informing and influencing, at emotional and intentional levels, our actions in reality (in this, he somewhat anticipated the discovery of mirror and canonical neurons, see Gallese and Umiltà, 2002; Gallese, 2007). This suggests that

> in his unconscious, Man is already a social animal genetically equipped with emotional structures that unconsciously prearrange and organise the acquisition of cultural codes. . . . Man is run through by an internal form of language of which he consciously grasps only a limited number of messages in the form of emotions—joy and pain, pleasure and displeasure—and of which he ignores the underlying, genetically preordained "grammar" or structure. Research into emotional codes is revolutionary because it originates from the study of the structure of linguistic codes and arrives at the living code, understood as the idiom of nature. In this way, a formidable means is created of restoring nature within culture. (Fornari, 1981, pp. 51, 280, translated for this edition; see also Gallese and Lakoff, 2005)

Fornari is well aware of the revolutionary character of what he proposes.

When Western Man began to suspect that our thought process might come from something that constitutes us from within, he drew upon the idea of a demon, or turned to the world of ideas, or of logical categories. The study of the living code instead represents a shift from the *world of ideas to the world of feelings*. Western theories of knowledge have been dominated by the relationship between the intellect and things in the outside world. . . . But we receive our naked thoughts directly from the living code in the form of feelings. The development of Western philosophical thought has forgotten that the sense of a subjective Self is founded on *a biological basis, which is even more material than socio-economic structures*. Furthermore, such a biological basis is primarily inhabited by the symbols of the living code which function as elemental metaphors of the living world. (Fornari, 1981, pp. 285–286; original italics, translated for this edition)

It is not easy to follow Fornari's language, but his intuition seems clear to me about a predominance of the "mental" in Western culture. Such predominance lead to positing an alleged superiority of rationality and to a historical devaluation of feelings, which are, instead, arguably essential to our being—reasoning and meaning making included—and cardinal to our existence in their power to orient us towards what is good for us and others.

Western culture has, instead, historically dealt with our affectivity only by demonising emotions as enemies of a mistaken notion of reason, reduced to a distorted and repressive rationality. This philosophical and moral framework has, accordingly, contributed to a complete disavowal of the reason of the body, of its feelings and emotions, in designing the ground rules for social life.

Fornari, to redress this "basic fault" of Western thought, advocates a return to a new form of humility against the hubris of our notion of a disembodied, illusionary mind, in recognising our dependence on a genetic prescription "of a natural code of signification" that "allows us to familiarise the world". He states that there is something "sublime" in this epiphany. Indeed, if we let ourselves really consider how we are pervaded in the very way we make meaning of our experience of being by such an all-comprehensive biological meaning-making code predisposing us for survival, I feel we cannot but be overwhelmed by awe and wonderment.

To generate affection, dreams and thoughts, the living code, being unsaturated, needs to meet with *an historic experience originally given by the mother and father*. We could then say the living code is the link

between nature and history. (Fornari, 1981, pp. 286–287; original italics, translated for this edition)

In other words, the genetic, neurobiological prescription predisposes,
but it also requires an encounter with an environment capable of
attuning to it on the same wavelength as the demand, to then meet it,
saturating it with its presence and resonance.

Fornari was not a neurobiologist, and neither am I. His reflections
stemmed from clinical work, where causes can be traced, following
the path inscribed by the pain of misattunements, all the way to the
primary offence that environmental deprivation inflicted on the physiology of emotions. Contemporary neuroscience substantiates the idea
of the living code by its discovery of epigenetic prewired action-
preparedness (Marcus, 2004). Fornari's ideas also find support in
recent studies in anthropology and ethology that suggest an idea of
evolution as a progressive dynamic characterised, as the complexity
of the species grows, by a motion towards a continuous and gradual
achievement of social cohesion. In other words, evolution would
proceed towards fostering a greater degree of relationships of cooperation and solidarity; this emergent tendency, thereby, would not only
have an ethical basis, but an evolutionary one, as it enhances the
survival potential of both the individual and the group. According to
this view, the fittest would not, therefore, be the strongest in terms of
muscle and brute force, but the one who enjoys a greater security
stemming from the empathetic support of his co-specifics and an
adaptive relationship with the environment. Moreover, this felt,
embodied sense of security would not only be a moment-to-moment
phenomenon, but also an internalised one, established in memory
through experience, allowing for a growth of autonomy and self-
reliance among individuals of phylogenetically higher species. In fact,
from an evolutionary standpoint, evidence suggests that survival has
been advantaged for species able to rely on the interdependence of
the individual and its co-specifics, as opposed to the ones driven by
opportunistic infra-species dynamics; and if this empathic ability,
which appears to mark the passage from lower mammals to primates,
represents one of the cornerstones of a child's maturation through the
recognition of the separation of the self from the other as an intentional agent, then it can be stated that morality has a solid neurobiological basis (Bertirotti, 2008, 2009; Damasio, 2008; de Waal, 1996;
Lorenz, 2002; Tinbergen, 1951; Tomasello, 2009).

Changes in treatment

> Without a reasonably valid theory of psychopathology, therapeutic techniques tend to lack precision and show uncertain benefits. Without a reasonably valid theory of aetiology, they will never receive the support of systematic and agreed-upon measures of prevention. (Bowlby, 1988, p. 37)

Such a shift in the understanding of the origins of psychic suffering necessarily calls upon us to radically rethink our therapeutic framework. Taking on board the physiology of human psycho-emotional templates fostering the fulfilment of survival-based needs, the core of treatment can in fact no longer be the futile attempt to adapt emotional needs to ill-devised social constraints, but must start from the recognition of the importance of an adequate environmental response, a response that first of all respects and understands the need itself. Thus, any therapeutic intervention has to start from an acknowledgement that there must have been an inadequate response in the history of the person who is suffering. The core of treatment, then, must focus on offering a relational opportunity that becomes therapeutic to the extent that it provides a meeting of those irreducible needs that have been thwarted: a meeting which the suffering person has long hoped for but never actually enjoyed; a meeting, furthermore, capable of restoring a disavowed part of the client's Self—all the more laden with pain and longing the more it has been denied—whose desperate request to be heard has been ignored and hidden for too long. "Everyone who was deprived of love as a child will long for it, sometimes their whole lives" (Miller, 2006, p. 204).

In order to comply to this reparative and integrative task, Fairbairn and Winnicott—aside from the different nuances in their theories—both suggest a therapeutic stance of empathic holding, which, together with the working through of repressed childhood experiences, may be capable of offering different and more appropriate emotional responses to the feelings of dismay, anguish, and solitude the client has suffered in childhood; the goal, for both theorists, is to provide a reparative experience of good object relationships that the person has not been provided with and which, therefore, are still missing in his or her internal world. According to both theorists, in fact, it is this lack that forms the origin of stilted emotional development, as well as of the distortion of the client's experience of her Self and needs.

In other words, from the standpoint of this new clinical framework, the therapist takes it upon herself to restore the "libidinal" through her holding and attuned response. The needy part of the client's self that was dissociated early on has, in fact, preserved its ability to grow, if freed from fear and terror, once a safe place to experience love can be found.

With regards to this, Bowlby speaks of a hidden "persistent potential for change", expressed through symptoms and leading to therapy.

> In providing his patient with a secure base from which to explore and express his thoughts and feelings the therapist's role is analogous to that of a mother who provides her child with a secure base from which to explore the world. The therapist strives to be reliable, attentive and sympathetically responsive to his patient's explorations and, so far as he can, to see and feel the world through his patient's eyes, namely to be empathic . . . A patient's way of construing his relationship with his therapist is not determined solely by the patient's history: it is determined no less by the way the therapist treats him. (Bowlby, 1988, pp. 140, 141)

A "cold" and "unsympathetic" response would, in contrast, inevitably preserve the status quo, reaffirming the inadequate parental behaviour that generated the problem in the first place: "were that so, the exchange would be anti-therapeutic" (Bowlby, 1988, p. 154).

Along similar lines, Miller claims that there can be no cure if ambivalence and healthy rage towards historically inadequate parental figures is not liberated from the feelings of guilt and "absolved": without a reappraisal of these strong childhood emotions it is impossible to allow feelings to finally move freely towards the building of healthy relationships in the client's present. Naturally, this is not so much a matter of "acting out" the aggression—more likely to occur when disavowed emotions are being ignored—but, rather, about using the therapeutic relationship to introduce a different template of response, one more receptive to, and attuned with, the patient's primary needs. A reparative experience of true meeting in fact spontaneously leads to a reorganisation of the client's experience of herself and of the world, which represents the premise on which it will ultimately become possible for the client to create healthy emotional conditions in real life. The experience of therapeutic holding intervenes where, in the very beginning, the original emotional response was lacking, failing to saturate the client's infantile emotional needs. Interposing the internalised memory of misattunement, the therapist can then provide the response that should have produced, at the start of the client's life, the development of the trust that allows imagining a world with baseline satisfactory relationships and establishes faith in one's own capacity to conquer them.

Therefore, the necessity to work through one's own history and to dare to look into failures in our earliest environment remains paramount to affect change. This is a necessary process meant to owning what actually happened, not placing blame, since, as Bowlby recalls, "the misguided behaviour of parents is more often than not the product of their own difficult and unhappy childhood" (1988, p. 145).

Therapy provides a setting with the potential to break the transgenerational and interpersonal transmission of insecure patterns of relatedness, as the work of taking our emotional wounds into awareness and repairing them interrupts the automatic repetition of traumatic exchanges. The attainment of healthy object relationships can change the course of existence, not only for the client, but also for his offspring (present or to come), in a direction more favourable to the enjoyment of life. Certainly, the therapeutic task is not an easy job, as those who suffer have learned to expect an attitude of persistent rejection. This was, in fact, the stance with which their childhood needs were actually received and, having internalised it, they learned to treat their emotional needs in the same way; our fragility is so great when we are little that the need for a reference point is such that a connection with bad objects is preferable to the total absence of objects. Once internalised, that rejecting or intrusive external object becomes an internal bad object, in whose attack the personality is still gripped.

As Winnicott suggests, it is necessary to recover the "real Self", an intimate and secret part of each and every one of us, the vessel of a vital energy. In our clients' stories, however, this lively subjective potential, not having been met, has been unable to express itself, but, rather, has had to adapt and remain secretly hidden, as if waiting for a moment in life when it could finally show itself and give rise to that process of growth, development, and self-expression that had been obstructed. Fairbairn says,

> The relationship existing between patient and analyst is more important than the technical details; and I would say the role of the analyst is not simply to perform the dual function of a screen, onto which the patient can project his fantasies, and a neutral instrument of interpretational techniques, but that his personality and motivations greatly contribute to the therapeutic process. (Fairbairn, 1957)

From the standpoint that there exists "a psychological basis for mental disorder . . . that it is possible to establish a clinical link between infant development and the psychiatric states, and likewise between infant care and the proper care of the mentally sick" (Winnicott, 2014, p. 158), the analyst is called upon to treat the patient's childhood aspirations as healthy parts. "*A belief in human nature and in the developmental process exists in the analyst* if work is to be done at all, and this is quickly sensed by the patient" (Winnicott, 2014, p. 292, original italics). First of all, Winnicott advises, the analyst must not be depressed, but instead be capable of offering an attentive ear, trust, and support without imposing any rules liable to foster premature adaptation into false identities based on complacency.

The therapeutic process thus becomes not only a release and compensation in the personal life of the client, but also a factor fostering social change by providing the means of releasing new emotional resources, finally legitimised and met, as part of an inherited history. Within the historic and biological evolution of society, these finally freed hidden potentials, once released, can in fact be deployed to change those social constraints responsible for the trauma in the first place.

Therapy thereby ceases to be a force fostering adaptation, as we realise that environmental failure at meeting human needs stems from social norms (embodied, in turn, in caregiving responses, and not only in the family) that have become sclerotic and actually prevent the promotion of useful, necessary conditions for the survival of the species and a better quality of relational life.

These considerations presuppose great awareness on the part of therapists and anyone with responsibilities in treatment or education, so as to avoid recreating situations of submission or complacent adaptation—easily tolerated by anyone accustomed to enduring them in their early childhood. I believe anyone in a nurturing role should instead fully comprehend the importance of rethinking the dominant values in our world if we want to start a process of spiritual renewal in our society, one that could save it in the first place.

If I insist so much on the need to transform the way treatment is designed, this is because I believe it is fundamental to understand that what allows the restoration of wounded emotional potentials—and with these also the ability to be truly *alive*—can only be an emotional response that reintroduces the hard-wired natural biological model of responsivity at the basis of secure relatedness. Understanding that affective experience is naturally as well as biologically structured in a patterned selection of psycho-emotional templates means extending to the world of our subjective experience the twentieth century's discovery that energy is always organised when it becomes matter. It follows that the momentum that feeds human life cannot be an impersonal flow seeking an aimless discharge, but it must be equally organised, and we have sufficient evidence today to claim that its emergent structure lies within bio-psycho-emotional and relational templates that guarantee and sustain our survival.

Psychoanalysis has insisted a great deal on the maternal figure, and rightly so, because everything inevitably begins from there. Emphasis has also been placed, though maybe not enough or not clearly enough, on how the maternal, as a symbol of return, release, and refuge, is, to some degree, never overcome. A constant need for regression—in the sense of secure surrender and release within a trustworthy holding environment—accompanies us throughout our lives, and not in any way as a sign of pathology. Freud's student and contemporary, Sándor Ferenczi, underscores, in his book *Thalassa* (1968), the importance of maternal rootedness in our lives, and writes at length about a "tendency to regression which governs both psychic and organic life" which finds expression, for instance, in sleeping or love-making, both subconscious expressions of a desire to return to bonding with the maternal body (Ferenczi, 1968, p. 83). So, according to the constitutive physiological tendency, the person should healthily "oscillate" between enjoyment of individuality and a need for a return to the release that this rootedness allows. As with childbirth, well-being therefore lies in a dynamic balance between the need for secure relational embrace and the one for individuation, moving between the security of an emotional known and the excitement of the unknown. Ferenczi wisely distinguishes this physiological need from those cases in which regression appears instead to be a sign of pathology, an obstacle to reaching maturity.

Bowlby, too, denounces the exclusively negative idea of dependence traditional to our culture, as if preserving and renewing the feeling of security experienced in secure attachment with the caregiver were necessarily pathological. We should, rather, highlight that pathological regression appears only in those histories marked by an unchecked prevalence of the maternal template caused by an absence—physical or emotional—of the paternal one, which instead could have provided a balance in its intrinsic fostering of autonomy.

It has to be noted that psychoanalytical thought has traditionally been partial in emphasising the importance of the maternal figure, going as far as theorising birth as a sort of trauma, almost as if life and autonomy were not gifts, and sanity relied on nothing more than a depressive working through of separation and loss.

In reality, the maternal world is no more omnipotent than anything else in life. The feminine needs the complementarity of the masculine—the encounter of the two is not by chance the basis of life—to provide the healthy nurturing environment needed by children to reach emotional maturity. If the mother is the "secure base" that permits trust and the illusion of perfect completeness at the beginning of life, the father is outlined secondarily on the child's experiential horizon as the precious companion allowing for secure exploration and invention. The father is the first and irreplaceable beacon, under whose affirming gaze the child can venture in the universe of emancipating activities, stimulating the acquisition of competence. The living proof of a security in being and doing, the father stands as the first example of autonomy and of external capability outside the maternal domain. With father alongside, one can dare. I think that, just as a woman is biologically supported and directed both neurologically and hormonally to perform her task with passion, so is the male, naturally equipped with less marked feminine parts and biologically orientated towards exploration and invention. Men are, therefore, just as fundamental in their caring role in encouraging the child's propensity to grow, supported in this task, we recall, by the maternal masculine, which gradually but inexorably, as in childbirth, scaffolds the child's emancipation from dependence.

I remember one of my own children, still in nappies and with a dummy in his mouth, spying on me from the doorstep of the kitchen as I was busy cooking to be sure of my presence, appearing to think "thank goodness you are here" before turning right back to whatever game he was playing. He stopped to look at me from the doorstep once and said, "You know, mummy, I was up there . . . I looked down and saw you and I said . . . I like that mummy there, and I came over." This made me understand that he felt his attachment for me still had an element of freedom in his detailing his judgement of me as the suitable mother for him. As if to say, "I came because you are this way, otherwise I would leave". He was defending his individuality, despite all the affection he felt for me.

The child's dual necessity, the need to be rooted as well as the need for autonomy, must therefore *both* be understood and protected. This also pertains to a mixture of masculine and feminine in terms of education and responsibilities. Growing up is hard without a model that accompanies and encourages; it is difficult to dare in a healthy way without someone willing to define for the child the boundaries that border the safe space for exploration—encouraging a child's freedom, while educating him to respect the rights of others.

The dual presence of the maternal and paternal code is also essential in therapy. If the revolution that occurred in post-Freudian psychoanalysis led to the re-evaluation of the need for empathic holding and for the authenticity of the therapeutic relationship (the only effective base for rebuilding that basic trust which is essential for coping with life), this must be intertwined with the therapist's willingness to guide and mark those boundaries that preserve life and its quality. This is a perspective clients alone often cannot see, unable as they are to sense, or allow themselves, the new experience of an emotionally available, empowering father. I think that psychoanalysis has all too often exclusively concentrated on regression, looking for dark areas of the unconscious, unduly prolonging treatment without bothering to offer patients the necessary reparative imprinting of secure relatedness which may fill the void, be internalised, and create the capacity to go out into the world and form meaningful, nourishing relationships. Indeed, often the offended childhood parts, those that need to be recognised and treated, have been cruelly interpreted as undue claims for a return to the maternal, as if something different were possible for someone who has never been able to fulfil the desire for symbiosis due to lack of adequate support at the right time.

Among classic psychoanalysts, Jung was perhaps the greatest advocate of the importance of the paternal archetype, even though, for personal and cultural reasons, he never fully developed his insights in this direction. He was, therefore, overall incapable of sufficiently underlining the importance of the father role as the architect of a healthy separation from the maternal world (Ferliga, 2005).

More recently, a number of authors have begun writing of the developmental damages provoked by an absence of the father figure which by many has been considered the leading cause of many serious psychic disorders that characterise our day and age. I believe, however, we must consider how this state of things is also the result of a radical transformation in our society and its daily habits, not just fathers' fault. At a social level, the Industrial Revolution in fact gradually made the traditional occupations of working the land or artisanship obsolete. These were for centuries the main activities performed by mankind, often shared with children, where

> the father passes on to the son a male know-how made of gestures, words, and silence, and the son's instinct is fed by the father's. Even daughters can watch their father as he works, and they see him at least at meal times. Thus, they develop an idea of the male figure that will accompany them their entire lives. Instead, the process of industrialisation kept the father figure away from the family the entire day, and put an end to this transmission of knowledge and experience, typical of pre-industrial societies based on farming and artisanship. With the waning of this transmission of traditions, much of male knowledge has been lost in both its physical and psychological dimensions. (Ferliga, 2005, p. 28, translated for this edition)

Moreover, in the twentieth century, two world wars removed the father figure for long periods of time, if not forever.

> After the terrible tragedy of the wars, first the economic recovery and later the development of consumer society kept fathers away from their children. Now the big multinational companies are responsible for kidnapping often complacent adult males from their families. In contemporary society, the man more frequently confuses his own fulfilment with the possibility of getting rich, willing to neglect his own children for work. He does not know or want to know how much pain this causes them. ... In this long process, begun by the Greeks five centuries before Christ, the father loses all his functions: pedagogical, spiritual, emotional, and as a generator of meaning. In the end, his only function is the one of the breadwinner, and his value is no longer measured by his qualities as a father, but by the depth of his pockets. (Ferliga, 2005, p. 32, translated for this edition)

Unfortunately, in contemporary society, not only the father figure has gone missing: the father's absence is in fact often joined by the mother's, equally forced by the social and economic system to work long hours that are incompatible with adequately taking responsibility over our young children's need for attachment and care.

In this regard, I find Brazelton and Greenspan's proposal for a "charter" of the seven irreducible needs of children fascinating. They suggest that such a scale could effectively be used to measure the level of civilisation of a nation instead of the usual, and often qualitatively meaningless, GDP. The two authors, moreover, raise their concerns over the fact that "institutional love" increasingly substitutes for direct childcare at the expense of the uniqueness and stability of an attachment figure the child so strongly needs.

What counts is not only the quantity, but also the quality, of care bestowed on the child. Neglect, in creating emotional deprivation, has effects just as catastrophic as food deprivation or the absence of a physically healthy environment.

> Providing for the irreducible needs of infants and young children and their families is the first step in producing citizens of a world who can broaden their sense of humanity sufficiently to cope with the new interdependency of the world

which can only be sustainable if based on respect and cooperation. However,

> we can't experience the consistency and intimacy of ongoing love unless we've had that experience with someone in our lives. (Brazelton & Greenspan, 2001, p. 182)

In other words, we cannot feel, propose, and spread emotions and healthy modalities of relatedness that we have never experienced, so the imprinting of secure, respectful, and collaborative relatedness must be protected in childhood. The economic system should, accordingly, understand that in order to have motivated workers, their need to provide care and attention to their children must be respected, through whatever means possible: flexible hours, part-time, or reduction of work hours. We must work in this direction, if we have even the vaguest idea of the importance of this change to ensure our survival as a species.

Recognition of emotional needs, however, finds a difficult reception, as it implies overcoming the exclusively competitive, productive viewpoint that has dominated our society. "Could our need to deny vulnerability in ourselves mean that we have to deny seeing it in our children?" (Brazelton & Greenspan, 2001, p. xix). There are actually reasons for great concern regarding the future of a society in which adults, having suffered deprivations in their youth, do not know how to feel and regulate their attachment needs. A society, thus, where people are never able to develop those emergent human characteristics, such as empathy and cooperation, which guarantee the possibility of serene and participatory social relations. I believe that emotional education should become a matter of specific studies alongside history, geography, or mathematics, if we want to be in time to compensate and rebalance the widespread ignorance regarding our human basic needs.

An invitation to change

We can do no more than "recognize that the environment created by our economic and social system, founded on the fragmentary and reductionist Cartesian worldview, has become one of the main threats to our health" (Capra, 1984, p. 266).

The study of the factors underlying physiological growth and pointing to an ecology of the mind has however appeared so far unable—as much as ecology in general—to make itself heard and warn a system that carries on convinced of being "the best of possible worlds". I wonder at what point we must arrive for the world to become aware that "civilisation" as we know it never took into account certain *fundamental* aspects of survival, having taken a view of Man that was unable to fully give justice to our nature in all its complexity. Nowadays, we can understand and study hitherto unexplored areas of the mind, but our economic and social organisation must really start and take this new knowledge into account if we are to avoid the threat of extinction, be it caused by the current disease of the planet or the just as severe malady stemming from our human nature's disavowal. The physical and emotional conditions in which we live become less liveable with every passing day, and require an epochal change. We have the means to do so, if only we are willing to think.

> Now that humanity finds itself in the midst of a planetary crisis, I declare myself *apocalyptic*, if this is what is called someone who thinks that, despite the *mortal crisis* we are experiencing, it still depends on us to act in such a way so that the outcome is not fatal. (Naranjo & Houston, 2007, p. 18, original italics)

Today, we know that quality and quantity of relatedness and exchange with the environment are both necessary elements for the survival and full development of our offspring. Widespread psychological suffering is the increasingly frequent sign, already grasped by Freud early on, of the decline of a civilisation. It is the crisis of a way of life that leaves no room for emotions, debasing and neglecting them, forgetting that the human brain, in its cognitive and emotional potential, initially develops only within a loving relationship capable of providing security. In its extreme economic development, our society has yet isolated and silenced the feminine and its reference to our childhood neediness. We have had the hubris of believing them superfluous, useless hindrances, without understanding that without them there can be neither life nor survival. It is not just women and children who are underestimated, considered partial objects to be forged into something useful for the system, it is also the feminine as a mental attitude that has been shunned; it is the emotional, the vulnerable, the frail, the playful, the ingenuous, of their own child-within, who has been extinguished and humiliated. People, men and women alike, live in denial of their own emotions and the child-within, even though these are just as much a part of everyone's nature, experience, history, and legacy, present in every human being, albeit in a unique mixture of tones and shades. There are those who speak of a necessary decline of the overly extended patriarchy in our history and culture. I do not see the crisis we are experiencing as the defeat of the "male", but more like the crisis of a distorted, hypertrophic "masculine" that has lost sight of the "feminine": believing society can do without its own intuitive side, its own right brain, to understand and approach the world. I believe the challenge we face is about restoring the balance between the two biologically wired poles and integrating them, because this is the only way, in the development of children as well as the development of society, to appraise the entire horizon of life.

From the practical standpoint, really taking on board what the study of mental distress has taught us in the twentieth century requires a correction in our value system, a critical reassessment of our working hours, an end to our fitful insistence on growth exclusively. Greater economic experts than myself have already argued along these lines (Latouche, 2004; Pallante, 2005; Sen, 1987, 1997; Shiva, 1988).

Do not tell me this is not possible. Mankind has beaten much greater odds when it came down to survival. We only need to want this, but to want something one must first understand. Something is certainly happening, perhaps the effect of the spreading worldwide crisis, as the recent financial repercussions are only the more superficial aspect of a much deeper and generalised betrayal of basic human needs. These also include the need for justice, respect, and fair trade. Among this suffering humanity, in such need of a healthy emotional integration, we are beginning to see some rare examples of alternative thinking. The task of filling the voids created by culture cannot be entrusted exclusively to therapists. Any society unable to deal with these voids, always accompanied by that specific suffering which lies at the root of aggressive and antisocial behaviour, is destined to perish. It is not enough merely to have children; parents must be able to care for them and nature dictates the ways and means of this care. This is not an option; it is a necessity that cannot be manipulated, transformed, or compressed to fit our lifestyles. Quite the contrary, it is society, with its organisation, that must respect nature and conform to those conditions that alone can guarantee its survival and quality.

Repression and the consequent neglect of our attachment needs create a state of permanent emotional instability. Although, on the one hand, this is useful to the system as it encourages consumption—presented and used in vain as compensation for needs that are much deeper yet denied—on the other hand, this produces a growing number of false adults absolutely incapable, both intellectually and morally, of assuming responsibility in whatever field they exercise their power. Just consider the seemingly infinite scandals that accompany political life: the superficial, inconsiderate choices behind the recent wars, the inability to organise the global economy more equitably and take political power away from serving big financial interests, and, finally, the hypocritical and ambiguous policies targeting the growing number of dispossessed in the world. There seem to be no responsible adults on the horizon capable of prudently leading society towards a balanced approach to real human needs. Meanwhile, a great multitude of citizen-children is parked in front of the television, distracted by sports events and shows, cheated with exhibitions of false happiness, spoiled with superfluous objects in the secret hope that they never grasp the fact that they actually have every right to claim the attention and respect which they have never received from those who present themselves as their leaders.

> Since those responsible for world affairs are more interested in appearances than they are in the essence of things, and more in details than fundamental aspects, only now have we reached a more general understanding of how the unhappiness in our condition is closely linked to lack of self-esteem and the repression of instinctive life. (Naranjo & Houston, 2010, p. 20)

So, change we must. Otherwise, I am afraid our final destruction will not be caused by an ecological disaster linked to the end of oil reserves or to the greenhouse effect. Long before any of that happens, in fact, psychological suffering, already widespread in the Western world, will seal the tragedy of a social organisation that is supremely disrespectful towards our basic biological needs as a species. A sociocultural, political, and economic system that, with its short-sighted knowledge and rules, has alienated the full enjoyment of life for everyone and created destructive relationships between individuals. A society, in short, less and less compatible with our survival.

CHAPTER FIVE

An emotional outlook on motherhood, or: what can really be done?

So, if psychology is really about the understanding of our emotional world and its needs, of how their dynamic balance stands at the basis of our survival and of the quality of our existence, we must conclude that it is an unknown science for most people. Everybody knows at least something about mathematics, sciences, languages, and history, but nothing is known about our emotional needs, about the need to securely attach and to be our own self. This, despite the existence of over a century of psychological literature whose development and results are now undisputed. This state of things, I believe, is also due to the fact that when we speak of emotional needs, we think of something natural and instinctive, which in theory is or should be true; however, we forget that in today's world the social and economic organisation within which we live, and which has primed our emotional responses and meaning-making, is far from any naturalness. Indeed, it seems designed more to ignore and repress it than to foster the expression of our natural makeup. Part of the responsibility clearly rests with the so-called experts who tend to limit their discussions to a closed circle of insiders, neglecting any attempts at effectively communicating to the world in accessible terms the fundamental elements of our findings. These, on the contrary, I believe should be available to everyone so that they may become a collective tool for living better, besides psychology's own (and crucial) contribution towards social improvement and progress. Even more unfathomable is the number of those who have no notion of evolutionary psychology or of the extraordinary discoveries in the more recent field of neurobiology, which confirm human beings' absolute necessity for relatedness. This is especially pertinent in childhood, when the need for secure and trustworthy emotional and capacitating references is paramount.

Alarmingly, the ranks of the uninformed include doctors and paramedics who work in hospitals with all types of patients: paediatricians who treat the physical health of children, obstetricians, social workers, but also teachers, who deal with children and adolescents on a daily basis. All these jobs have profound emotional significance and require knowledge about healthy attachment patterns and the ability to offer them.

This, obviously, not to mention parents. Parents are currently bombarded with all sorts of theories, or, even worse, urged on with feigned wisdom by their own relatives, who often interfere intensively and intrusively in the care to dictate rules on the basis of their alleged educational expertise. These inputs are useful only for disorientating parents. Surrounded by a world of advertisements that seduce them with flattering messages, aimed only at making them faithful consumers, parents are today totally lacking a source of information that can explain to them the crucial role they play and the poetry of their function. Only understanding their role in terms of meaning, rather than a list of confusing and anxiety-provoking instructions, can help parents cope with the demands of their commitment and effort with the certainty of a guidance, both internal—prepared for by their own emotions—and external, that can accompany and empower them in making their babies into children and, later, serene and contented adults.

As I argued before, it would also be worthwhile if politicians and economists were made aware of the new discoveries in psychology, so that, instead of being attentive only to growth and development, or worried only about satisfying this or that group in a constant hunt for votes and consensus, they might also pay some attention to the needs of those who cannot speak for themselves but who represent the men and women of tomorrow. Children now and future capable members of society in the future will be all the more happy and accomplished, in fact, if the social and economic system provided the appropriate conditions for their care, growth, and education.

The observation of this "not-knowledge" was what surprised me the most when I first came into contact with the world of maternity. Coming from the new psychiatric movement, this was a new setting for me and this unexpected "ignorance" of their patients' (and their own) emotional needs among the rest of the staff in the maternity ward was among the factors that compelled me to engage in it. I wanted to find a way to communicate and apply the knowledge I had gained from my studies as well as my experience from years of treating psychiatric patients—where, sadly, I had first-hand experience of the tragic effects of early environmental failures—so as to make good use of it as an effective means of prevention.

As I have already detailed, pregnancy is a period charged with biological and emotional meaning. I strongly believe that an affective reading and understanding of the wealth of messages bestowed by nature to childbirth can be more worthwhile than the study of an entire treatise in psychology. This is so if, naturally, by psychology we mean knowledge of the physiology of emotions and not exclusively the treatment of mental distress. I have never understood why, in the field of psychology, there is so little talk of health, as if, unlike physical well-being, nature had not expressed itself on the conditions that guarantee it very clearly.

I was fascinated by, and involved in, Fornari's attempts to devise a simple, yet effective, method of providing a "training in affectivity" to personnel in hospitals and public institutions who are daily involved with, and often engrossed in, relationships with patients—shadowing Balint's pioneering experience with general practitioners (1955). However, in my own experience in maternity wards, rather than a training through and through, I have found it more effective and meaningful to simply present colleagues with an account of birth in its emotional meanings and a narrative overview of the developmental pathway that takes the human affective world from the domain of symbiosis and childhood dependence to the achievement of adult exchange and reciprocity—as described here in Chapter Two. This I found to be the most immediate way to lead my colleagues, daily engaged in assisting pregnancies and births, to a comprehension of the underlying emotional weft of meaning, providing them with the means with which to grasp and interpret something that no one had previously taught them to read.

Therefore, the training I offered the staff of the maternity ward where I worked simply consisted in a developmental overview of the physiology of emotional growth. Starting off with a presentation of the historical and deeper meaning of our intrinsically symbiotic origins, I then dwelled on the embodied characteristics of the maternal, already expressed in pregnancy, as an emotional holding that contains but never withholds. I described the emotional meaning of labour, highlighting the crucial gradualness that needs to prepare the passage from passive to active symbiosis, and offered a reading of childbirth as an event that embodies the complementarity of feminine and masculine templates, establishing their parity as both fundamental for individual development and the survival of the species. I stressed the necessity of encouraging and protecting the bonding process so as to leave to the woman an active role in encouraging her child to attach, to then letting him to separate only when the time is right. I offered an interpretation of breastfeeding as an emotional experience that gradually leads to the newborn's discovery of relatedness, and proceeded to emphasise the presence of masculine and feminine templates in both sexes, although with different nuances. Finally, I explained how the dynamic interplay of these complementary templates is what creates the facilitative environment for a secure attachment and equally secure separation; finally I detailed how this integrated provision stimulates the child's unique potential of competence and aptitudes to emerge throughout the various stages that articulate and express the unfolding of a developmental process wherein hereditary factors will be epigenetically negotiated within environmental conditions.

As the reader can see, this is not a directive training that imposes or suggests rules of behaviour, which, in my opinion, prove totally useless, if not harmful, as rules hinder spontaneity in the way staff members relate to patients. My aim was, rather, to offer, with humility, my own emotional resonance to this awe-inspiring narration, calling upon the staff's own emotional response to this highly charged content; the story of human emotional birth, in fact, is the account of something that touches *everyone's* emotional experience, as it evokes an inevitable comparison with our own history as children. It has the power to signify, providing a meaning matrix to our memories and emotions; it makes us quietly reflect upon the care we received, encouraging an understanding of what eventually went missing, and it can validate our own suffering for not having experienced what we are hard-wired to expect and need so desperately: a loving, holding and capacitating care. I find that, although it appears to be just a lecture, it really is talking about ourselves, because each of us has been through the same experience. Furthermore, knowing about our coming into being, and the origins of the way we feel, is a way to become able to more accurately appraise others, while, at the same time, looking inside oneself; a way to reflect on one's own personal experience and understand, as I suggest, that the only way to comprehend other people's internal world is really to know one's own.

In providing this overview, I also always added a historical and scientific justification to my approach, just as I have done in this text. I in fact believe this is a useful premise so that everyone may understand the difficult emotional and cultural journey that we need to face and conquer if we want to dare think outside of the usual trite and limited conceptual patterns.

Often, people have been actually moved to tears by the story of how a human baby is born as a person, within the embrace of a relational matrix that holds and propels us to life. In consideration of the strong emotional charge of the content, being moved I find somewhat inevitable and even desirable, given that, either for generational or cultural reasons, everyone has his or her own skeletons in the cupboard. The important thing to understand is that the feelings we have are extremely valuable, as they reflect and give us back the truth of what we have experienced, and there is no reason to hide or to be ashamed over this. On the contrary, it can be quite useful. To be moved by this narration can in fact constitute a precious opportunity, a testament to how emotionality is an unavoidable part of our existence, our record-keeper, the bearer of our truth, an indicator of what we missed and need. Something that accompanies us, permeates our corporeity, providing us, the same way as our senses, with an embodied appraisal of the quality of the environment in which we move informing us on how to behave once we have "sniffed around": if we should trust or doubt, if we are attracted or afraid, if we are curious or uncertain.

This is a talk about emotions, but more than that. This is depicting them as the expression of a vital energy inherently organised in affective patterns: evolutionarily crafted clusters of needs, behaviours, attitudes, emotions, motivations, and expectations that are necessary and crucial for survival. Powers then, and not hindrances, useful instruments for finding our bearings and coping better with life by integrating in our awareness its appraisal through our feelings. More importantly, this is about making friends with those same emotions that a heedless culture and thoughtless science have labelled as dangerous and blind. This perspective in fact allows us to see maturity as the ability to let us make full use of our senses in construing our appraisal—integrating visceral and emotional feedback, internal and external, with our cognitive processing—to orient our actions and inform our decision making—something a child can learn only by having a caring adult model. This thereby conveys that, contrary to what our culture taught us, intelligence does not lies in the triumph of a blind, vulgar rationality, which represses feelings and is, thus, condemned to move without an appraisal of what is truly valuable.

As the reader can see, the presentation never willingly enters the personal, but aims to represent and outline the physiological movement of affections in their process of maturation from dependence to reciprocity as a paradigm. It can be fascinating to discover that no energy in nature is disorganised, not even emotional energy, and that it is up to we humans—as opposed to animals, who do it instinctively—to choose and adhere to the relational modality best suited to the circumstances we experience. This perspective implies, in fact, that becoming an adult cannot be considered the conquest of a granite, a-contextual, self-sufficiency—whenever we find this, in fact, it is a bad sign—but that secure maturity instead remains a continuous oscillation between a prevailing modality of reciprocal exchange and the reappearance of more child-like modes of dependence in which the need for abandon and trust can be met and savoured anew; it is allowing for this very oscillation that actually fuels the adult desire to express this both as recipient and as provider for others in need. Childhood is, therefore, never fully outgrown. An indelible part remains in both our memories and our emotional outlook on life; child-like aspects of our deep sensitivity are, in fact, custodians of our curiosity and creativity, but also of our fragility and weakness, a companion in our pleasure in expressing ourselves and in our constant need for affection.

As we discussed, this form of training can touch upon the personal sphere, present and past, of the audience. There are those who are more inclined and those less inclined to let it evoke personal experiences, and that is perfectly all right. Nevertheless, I find that access to emotions is facilitated if they are represented as healthy natural forces, guiding our appraisal of reality and our behaviour towards that saturation of our needs that underlines well-being. Our emotional responses, moreover, give us an instant experience of being-in-time, tied as they are to the circumstances in which one has grown; they are, thus, useful means of facilitating reflection and an understanding of oneself and others. It is easier to learn to cope with feeling if, in a group—where the intersubjective and relational holding makes it more secure—one accepts to put their emotions into play without hesitation and learns to interpret through them the emotional environment which one is called to respond.

By looking more closely, one can see that one of the motives that forces people into hiding their emotions is the idea that they are not legitimate. I tend to believe—as is also suggested by Alice Miller (1983, 1990, 2006) or neurobiology, which places it in the deep memory area of the limbic system—(Siegel, 2012; Siegel & Hartzell, 2003), that the so-called unconscious is not an entity, but, rather, that it is constituted by the processes and contents making up our autobiographical (embodied and experiential) memory. This, deposited in our brains, appears to as a historical–dynamic agglomerate capable of reaching our consciousness only if culture permits and facilitates such passage, and if the resurfacing of memory does not endanger the individual's emotional balance. The notion that our emotional responses are illegitimate or shameful, therefore, stems from a culture and common thought that exercises a veto, making us feel guilty and returning us to that feeling little in fear of losing approval. All the same, as time goes by, what was unmentionable in Freud's time is altogether much less unspeakable today, and I think that even what Miller sees as an insurmountable problem—the courage to denounce parents' mistakes in child-rearing—can simply become a sad but understandable fact of general awareness. We now know, in fact, and have the empathy to understand, that failures in care stem not from evil parents, but from the very human limitations of those who preceded and influenced us, due to a general non-knowledge. This can be remedied by sharing and confessing the pain, which, in turn, can release the resources to implement change so that those who come after us may suffer less than we did.

In this sense, we can say that the 1968 student protest movement—with all its limitations, contradictions, exaggerations, and impatience—did indeed manage to introduce a deep shift in collective awareness. This is because, at the root of the many particular demands of that time, there was implied a revolution in the way of thinking: a liberation from atavistic clichés, a new-found courage to dream—not as mere evasion, but as an anticipation of a real possibility for change. The effects of this epochal change in sensibility, admittedly through alternate phases of proposal and fearful return to the status quo, we are only now beginning to enjoy. Even the election of Barack Obama as President of the United States of America, something unthinkable only a few years ago, shows how, through indescribable effort, humanity can hesitantly acquire the ability to renew itself when faced with the threat of annihilation.

As I was saying, not everyone reacts in the same way during staff training, but I have never heard a sarcastic or disrespectful comment on the subject matter I presented. I have often been called an idealist, a romantic, by colleagues, who then, however, went on to become affectionate companions in the experience of group supervisions in which they were more than happy to share in their burden of responsibility and care in treating difficult cases and receive emotional support.

Moreover, if we understand that it is fundamental for a child to be able to trust an adult, and that nature, with its neurobiological processes, sparks and establishes the child's primary attachment in the same way as it prepares a proper emotional response in the mother and father, then we can extrapolate from this natural model of care—not through simplification or trickery, but simply because this is the way it really is—the outline of a care template. This would befit all those situations, even in adult life, in which there is a momentary and passing need to be cared for and led, accompanied and escorted through an experience about which we feel worried and in need of someone more expert or more capable to act as our guide. The doctor–patient relationship is a stark example of such a case.

On the doctor's part, understanding the attachment-based counterparts of the care relationship involves an availability for a commitment which cannot be merely technical, but must also be emotional. And it is always preferable to be aware of this and its necessity, so as to better navigate these waters; otherwise, the risk is to lose, as is currently happening, all control of the situation while facing increasingly pressing demands. If this is generally valid for all fields of medicine, I believe it is even more important in the field of assisting pregnancy, which is not a medical event—unless of course there are complications for one reason or another—but primarily an emotional one, in which the woman, due to an important physical and emotional transformation, regresses to a state of heightened sensibility and fragility.

Therefore, in maternity in particular, assistance must be informed by a willingness to relate and feel as well as by medical expertise if it wants to be effective at passing on information and guidance. The ability to adequately relate from an emotional standpoint becomes, thereby, the best guarantee of building trust and, ultimately, the success of the process. In the medical debate, it is well known that often accidents or complications, on verifying the facts, turn out to have been caused more by incorrect communication than actual medical error. Once the emotional template inherent to the relationship of dependence is understood, the possibility rises to create a relationship capable of making people feel heard, which creates the trust needed to accept guidance. The care template in fact informs a form of accompanying without abusing power—a template capable of containing, guiding, and setting reassuring limits.

The medicalisation of pregnancy: how to move beyond it?

If pregnancy and birth are physiological aspects of existence, it is amazing that these events should have become so strongly medicalised that the majority of users end up having a sense of going through some sort of obstacle course, full of traps and pitfalls, to be run only with the escort and guarantee of a mighty (almighty?) medical figure to prevent otherwise inevitable failures.

Truth be told, this happens in all fields of medicine. It appears that many, in the modern day and age, seem to consider physiology something of a curiosity and submit to scores of sometimes useless (if not outright harmful) treatments seemingly just for reassurance, as well as proceed to anxiously integrate their intake of supplements and vitamins of doubtful efficacy with a range of over-the-counter products conveniently advertised as cure-alls.

In this sense, pregnancy is in good company. Any trust in its physiological and natural unfolding appears to have been all but disappeared, or, to be more accurate, confidence has been bestowed upon a myriad exams and check-ups that, in collective imagination, act as "magical" guarantees of success. Prenatal courses run by midwives, who should be the natural figures of reference for physiological pregnancies, have great difficulty taking off due to a widespread mistrust. Doctors, from this perspective, inspire more confidence, as if the process could not possibly succeed without medical aid. Furthermore, the rampant emotional immaturity that characterises service users these days makes them highly dependent on seeking constant guarantees and reassurance outside of themselves, often from a position of anxious and resentful entitlement. As our society deprives most people of the relational means to reach emotional maturity, a lot of adults are in fact grown-up only on the outside, whereas emotionally are still like children who had no way of building some form of self-assurance and trust in their own biological and emotional competence. This appears to me to be the underlying reason why medicine—which, in pregnancy, should be humbly integrated into the natural course of events and intervene only where absolutely necessary (and, in these instances, it does have real, often life-saving value!)—has invaded every single step of the way to motherhood. The sad counterpart of this state of things is that maternity, stripped of its deepest emotional meanings, looks more and more like the anxious setting for a service supply and demand pervaded by the implicit blackmail that, if something goes wrong, someone must be accountable. It has become a "business", and, unlike a therapeutic alliance between doctors and patients, we see the relationship between "consumers" and "medical providers" being marked by a denial of partaking in a natural process which, as is the case with all of life's events, carries an element of uncertainty and the possibility of failure. The implicit appeal to physicians is, thereby, an often despotic demand for a guarantee—bestowed by science—along with the unspoken threat of legal blackmail in case of failure. In this game, fed by a myopic and illusory quest for power, doctors pay heavily for their hubris, as insurance policies eat up their profits and their nights are made sleepless by anxiety.

Furthermore, colluding with the service users' subconscious demand for absolute certainty, recently we have witnessed the intrusion of other medical experts—including clinical psychologists—in the maternity "business", eager to do their best to smooth out complexities instead of seeking to understand them. We are, for instance, witnessing not only the medicalisation, but also the psychiatrisation, of motherhood. Consider the recently proposed assimilation of motherhood into post traumatic stress disorder (PTSD) (DiBlasio & Ionio, 2001; Maggioni et al., 2009) or the nationwide hunt for post-partum depression (PPD) as if it were a constituent and even inescapable part of the adventure of motherhood, best combated with tests and psychotropic drugs.

> An important aspect of the mechanistic concept of living organisms and the consequent engineering approach to health is the belief that the treatment of infirmity requires some form of external intervention on the part of the doctor ... taking into consideration the patient's potential for recovery. This attitude descends directly from the Cartesian concept of the body as a machine that needs repairing when it breaks down. ... In the process of reducing infirmity to a sickness, the attention of doctors shifts far from the patient as a whole person. ... Modern reductionist medicine ... has developed disciplines so specialized that frequently doctors are no longer capable of seeing in an infirmity a disturbance in the entire organism, nor treating it as such. (Capra, 1984, pp. 127, 131)

As I have written elsewhere, among the various transitions in life, pregnancy is perhaps the one most marked by an intense emotional meaningfulness. It is, indeed, a central passage in our existence, setting the boundary, for men and women, of the end of an era; it in fact hallmarks, physically and emotionally, the passage from being daughters and sons to becoming mothers and fathers, acquiring parental responsibility through the course of a biological process.

> The emotional significance of pregnancy ... its trademark anxiety, is what makes midwifery, which "treats" or simply accompanies its physiology, a "special" field of medicine. Its object, in fact, is not an illness, but an event charged with enormous emotional resonance. This means that, compared to other medical specialisations where the attachment relationship between doctor and patient is an important but not as central an element to comprehend, in midwifery the relationship *is* the object of the job. There is, thus, a special need for an attentive training so that health workers who are involved in supporting pregnant women and their partners can be made able to identify and facilitate the emotional physioloy that marks the unfolding of this wonderful process; and, on the other hand, learn to identify and

appropriately deal with any pathological deviation from the normative psycho-emotional pathway that might occur. (Mieli, 2003, p. 71,
translated for this edition)

Pregnancy is, therefore, a physical and emotional passage that,
even if desired and expected, inevitably entails a psychological working through, as it marks the passage of time and ages, whereby
parents-to-be are confronted with the task of facing the profound
mark of heritage and the embodied meaning of generational succession. A culture less in a hurry and less superficial than ours would
know how to celebrate and participate more harmoniously in the
different stages of life, and how to accompany the turmoil inherent
in this passage with more adequate emotional sharing. Pregnancy is,
indeed, a physiological upheaval, and, like all changes in life, it bears
the ambivalence of any process of becoming. Any change, in fact,
sees the joy of novelty chased by the mourning of a loss, with that
combination of curiosity and nostalgia, desire and melancholy that is
typical, as we have seen, of childbirth: daring and retreating, leaning
out and withdrawing fearfully; this is not a sign of pathology, but a
physiological pattern which marks any process of growth in life, an
oscillation whereby the safety of the known becomes a valuable tool
for comprehending and tackling the new.

For all these reasons, I believe that a strictly medical and technical
outlook risks underestimating and neglecting the emotionality
implicit in this momentous passage. Indeed, it feels almost as though
avoidance and disavowal of this difficult, yet necessary, working-
through were a prescription. Running away from it, in fact, we also
avoid the effort of questioning our cultural reductionism and of
embracing any more holistic views capable of keeping up with the
complexities of the event. And then we cry crocodile tears whenever
we end up reaping the consequences for not having heeded the warning signs when things go terribly wrong.

Throughout the years, the increasingly sanitised quality of the
relationship between patient and health-care professional has led to
a situation in which the knowledge and responsibilities of the doctor
have lost their role, while physicians live under the threat of legal
action at the whims of service users. I remember a top clinician and
obstetrics professor who participated with me at a convention where
I spoke about the affectivity that runs through pregnancy and
birth, and how it should be understood and managed. When it was

his turn to speak, he addressed me with self-importance and sarcasm: I was lost in romantic ideals—he argued—because what women really want is to book a Caesarean section. And you, Professor—I answered—play the requested song like a jukebox into which a coin has been inserted. The debate, however, unexpectedly shifted in my favour with the projection of some statistics and numbers derived from British data—considered by the medical community the best science could offer—whereby the professor found himself having to somehow justify the exception offered by the small town of Shrewsbury, Shropshire (which I knew well, since I had sent my children there to learn English) which, contrary to the national trend, showed a limited number of C-sections. The professor had eventually to admit that the quality of assistance offered there, marked by a strong celebration and passion that accompanied every newborn baby, may *perhaps* explain the data. I shall always remember this incident with fondness as "a triumph of emotional data".

As it has been argued, there is evidence that if all maternity ward staff were trained in the physiology of affectivity, it would also give them the means to usefully manage the relationships with patients. Such awareness in fact, could render them able to transform the course of a pregnancy from a series of check-ups and exams—which users often mistakenly attribute the power to magically influence, positively or negatively, the outcome—to an emotional event in which emotions, including fears and doubts, can be discussed because someone is interested in hearing them. It is very important that, especially during pregnancy, emotional signals are communicated to the medical staff. If the accompanying climate were an attuned one, it would be much easier for the woman to confide and share, receive attention and support, without feeling shame over her experience. If the care were organised along these lines, it would be conveyed to the woman that the road to motherhood is normally paved with emotions and uncertainties, and that only exchange with others can supply the answers to her questions and help her cope and regulate her feelings. This is the template of secure attachment. In the final analysis, it is better to ask questions than not to ask them. Voicing is proof of awareness and facilitates taking responsibility over what the visceral experience is signalling to us. The availability of emotional attention, therefore, already acts as a first level of prevention, since it facilitates the expression of feelings, creating a template of secure relatedness in sharing, and teaching one to love one's weaknesses and doubts instead of repressing them or refusing to acknowledge them as one's own. We all know that whatever we try to deny always finds some other way to be heard—sometimes a dangerous one.

Furthermore, if medical and obstetrical personnel were equipped to understand, expect, and facilitate the natural course of the emotional process underlying pregnancy, then they could easily identify situations in which the emotional tension transcends that physiological pathway. In fact, pregnancy can also be marked by emotions that go beyond the normal ebb and flow of feelings evoked by a project as loaded with expectations as this one. It is important to know that a degree of heightened emotionality is normal as, on top of the normative load of anticipation, the woman's increased emotional reactivity is also due to the hormonal modification that, as we have seen, is responsible for attuning a woman's sensitivity to that of her baby. This is so that she may more easily identify with his needs and act to their advantage, from the standpoint of the survival of the species, through the intense and precious bond between mother and child. We often hear of a pregnant woman's "regression." This is not an expression I like, because I fear it might be associated with the idea of an illness, when, instead, it refers to this physiological and useful transformation meant to facilitate good-enough mothering. This special emotional state was mentioned also by Winnicott and Bowlby, and before them by the only other psychoanalyst who focused specifically on pregnancy, Helene Deutsch. She, however, went a bit further, by recognising in this emotional alteration of the pregnant woman a valid justification for the emergence of sudden unexpected difficulties. This insight of hers makes her contribution salient, although today her *The Psychology of Women* (Deutsch, 1945) might seem a little naïve and prone to simplification due to its close adherence to Freudian structure. Nonetheless, it is true that in the emotional ride that takes the woman back to childhood, every mother-to-be returns to her own history and experience as a little girl. This direct contact with her emotions might hence bring back some remote experiences, together with memories: unexplored events and long-forgotten feelings that suddenly break into the expectant mother's consciousness, reawakened by the absorption in her emotional world that is pertinent to this period. So, it is only normal that if the personality's balance was only apparent or, at least, had been worked out at the expense of leaving some deep, early experiences unintegrated, it may be unexpectedly upset by this re-emergence of the past. The release of distress, in such instances, however, paves the way for the possibility of a new understanding, even of what had to be disavowed in the process of growing up.

Often, in my clinical experience, I found that it is these repressed emotional memories that really lie behind the fear of childbirth, or the fear of pain, the requests for scheduled C-sections, or the occurrence of certain sudden or inexplicably difficult deliveries. Disavowal is, unfortunately, also facilitated and encouraged by a climate of rampant, so-called "feminist" disinformation aimed at advertising the advantages of a painless delivery often spurred by the triumph of superficial word-of-mouth depicting childbirth as torture. This has, obviously, little or nothing to do with scientific information. Unfortunately, however, un-investigated, misunderstood difficulties in our world always find their prosthesis, eagerly provided by the law of the marketplace. However, a technical response to women's fear is not the answer if that technical fix is not grounded in understanding: a thorough understanding, one based on a scientific outlook on childbirth that has the courage to humbly explore its workings to understand it in all its splendid complexity. Otherwise, I often provocatively ask: What would we do with a starry sky, a fiery sunset, if we could get inside them and tame them? What is more fascinating about love than the feeling of being swept off one's feet by an emotion that surpasses any explanation or control? In offering a quick fix to women's fears not a single consideration in fact is made regarding the emotional course of pregnancy, while women themselves are not informed of the meanings behind their physiological manifestations, including labour pain. In prenatal courses, as we have said, little information is given regarding the emotional and relational aspects underlying motherhood. Positions, contractions, breathing, and breastfeeding are all discussed, but there is no introduction to the wonderful world of the mother–child relationship or any description of the meaning and function of the unfolding of the various stages before and after the actual delivery. As a matter of course, the mother or couple is told what to do, but not why, as no explanation or emotional foundation is offered that might give justice to the pleasure and emotion of parenthood. There is no unravelling of the important messages that nature aims to imprint and convey through the physicality of pregnancy and childbirth, and neither is any rationale provided as to why it is so paramount to yield to a pathway whose set points are embodied and emotional. Parents-to-be seldom have explained to them the crucial importance of fostering a renewed symbiosis during the postnatal period as a necessary foundation for the infant's renewed sense of security entraining his autonomic nervous system. No care is taken in providing a horizon of expectations, in explaining the slow mental and emotional evolution the newborn baby needs to perform, first through contact with his mother's body, then in an increasingly wider encounter with reality thanks to the mother's encouragement and the father's participation.

If these basic aspects of parenthood are not explained (and, in the light of current evidence, the availability of these emotional provisions to the child are no educational options but scientifically proved necessities), then it is as if couples were made to travel one of the most important journeys of their life without any road signs. And feeling lost ruins the pleasure of the ride because of the anxiety of not knowing. Clearly, in such insecure circumstances, as if advancing in the darkness of total uncertainty, any recipe peddled as easing or even erasing difficulties will be eagerly accepted. And the general public is not alone in falling for any passing fad; professionals do as well, spurred by the growing confusion due to *not knowing*.

In the prevailing of a culture as dismissive towards meanings as the one in which we live, the general preoccupation is simplification and the use of technology to rid the world from the oppression of all difficulty and exertion. What happens in maternity is, in fact, simply the extension of a more general attitude towards other difficult, but meaningful, aspects of life. And if science and technology work wonders in many fields—and we are grateful to them for it—on the other hand, their successes seem to have "gone to their heads", as they keenly pursue a fix-all role serving the goal of an impossible sugar-coating of human life, or the equally impossible goal of exceeding its constitutive boundaries. I am referring, for example, to pathetic attempts at rejuvenation that cannot cancel age; IVF allowing for pregnancies in conditions and at ages excluded by nature for good reasons; or the obsessive search for the perfect child by earlier and earlier diagnosis of disability; and, finally, to eugenic attempts through DNA tampering.

This only goes to show a generalised Western difficulty to refrain from the temptation of playing the almighty, a sad infatuation that vainly masks a deep, widespread inability to confront pain and limitations.

In the general readiness to adapt to a world where everything must be quick—painless, without emotion, "comfortable for oneself and screw the others", facilitating a surrogate of survival based on running and producing—then even pregnancy, childbirth, love, motherly and fatherly care, waiting, hoping, suffering, trepidation, patience, exhaustion, in short, life itself, runs the risk of transcending our own ability for comprehension and acceptance. We never ask ourselves, in this simplified version of existence, in this "reductionism" of living, if something is escaping us: not something superfluous but fundamental. This is the whole point. Because without emotions, in their alternating opposites, there is no life, and above all there is no mental health. So, knowing how to preserve them allows for a better life. (Mieli, 2003, p. 37, translated for this edition)

Here, I would argue, is where the claim is born to clear the difficult path of motherhood—and, therefore, of life itself—of all its constituent difficulties and uncomfortable aspects, obviously considering only the physical aspect of what we want to get rid of and not its significance. Science and technology eagerly step in to tackle and transform this natural event to make it more acceptable for women who want a simplified version of it.

Thus, we witness a disastrous chase that sees service users peremptorily requesting "civilised" facilitations more "appropriate" to the twenty-first century; while science, with medicine in first place, is eagerly prepared to go to great lengths to find adequate shortcuts for the modern woman. Too bad the emotional needs of children are still the same. No one seems to have considered that if nature organised childbirth in a certain way—evolutionarily crafted over millennia—there must be some reason. Nobody seems to wonder that perhaps there is a reason why the mother's womb takes so long to let go of its fruit, just as it makes sense that the child should stay in the womb for nine months and would do better not to come out early, or why it takes a lot of time, dedication, and commitment for a child to grow and, possibly, to grow well. Only a few enlightened paediatricians dare nowadays inform us of the advantages of natural childbirth in facilitating the gradual physical and emotional adaptation of the newborn baby to the new environment, which requires new abilities.

Nevertheless, it should not be surprising that, according to polls conducted after childbirth, almost no woman who underwent a C-section wants to repeat the experience. In my own work, I, too, encountered a keen sense of disappointment and deprivation in women who underwent a C-section. Catherine Dolto, daughter of the famous French psychoanalyst, has developed a body therapy framework, called haptonomy, to help Caesarean children through difficulties that appear to turn up punctually in their adolescence—a new birth—because of the loss of an active birth experience (Dolto, 1999).

The widespread fear of pain has created a new opportunity for anaesthesiologists, most of whom, curiously, are women, intent on devising refined new techniques to deliver women from such a "degrading" experience as labour. And even though the past few years have heard mostly talk of epidural anaesthesia, today the most widely circulated new product is a hypnotic drug called Ultiva, which completely pacifies the woman, not by acting on pain, but by fostering an estrangement from the live experience of childbirth.

Women are hardly made aware that drugs practically nullify all active participation, and with it all the enjoyment and appreciation of one's own competence and ability. All these trends turn the avoidance of pain into the central aspect of delivery, forgetting all mention of the deep sense of love and participation experienced in welcoming one's own child into life in the world.

Nevertheless, I hate ideologies that become slogans. I have never been a fan of all-natural childbirth at any cost, either. It is truly depressing to watch constantly conflicting ideologies become entrenched in their own excesses, one against the other, unable to reach any reasonable mediation.

I believe it would be enough to return to a concept of assistance as instrument for helping the woman. This could be easily integrated with a recognition of her suitably stimulated abilities, and with the physician and service user's shared knowledge and awareness that pregnancy and childbirth must be considered with respect and attention for their internal coherency of meaning and processes. In sum, the way forward should be just protecting and fostering the physiological pathway and its emotional substratum, rather than trying to ameliorate it with our intrinsically limited understanding of the complexity that permeates it.

Similarly, I have never been against the use of epidural anaesthesia when necessary, evaluated on a case by case basis; such as, for example, when neither preparation nor awareness, nor even the presence of an adequately attentive atmosphere, are enough to provide the necessary serenity for the successful separation of a child from his mother.

I am against it, instead, when the intention is to make it an unquestioned rule that must not be debated, so that it would seem strange for someone to want to avoid it. The theory behind such a degraded view is, in fact, that it is

> a facilitation for civility, an instrument capable of restoring a woman's dignity, saving women from the degradation of losing their cool: screaming, "animal-like", something so unbecoming these days. Everything is easier, calmer, under control, less of a "mess": so much the better . . . (Mieli, 2003, p. 35, translated for this edition)

Midwives know how important their emotional relationship is with the woman, in the best-case scenarios a relationship initiated during pregnancy. Experienced obstetricians know their role is all about "being there", helping the woman recognise and release her potential and energy, and make it through (Gaskin, 2003; Schmid, 1998, 2005, 2007, 2011). They also know a one-on-one relationship is preferable; it conveys commitment and implies the act of taking a personal and emotional responsibility in accompanying the woman through a challenging process while making her feel held through earning her trust by one's quality of *being there*. Trust, instead, is inevitably lost if there is a change of hands with a new shift and the new midwife has to restore it from scratch, if there is time.

The fear of childbirth—not a problem for every woman, regardless of common prejudice—in my professional experience always has profound justifications in her attachment history and certainly cannot be written off as mere fear of physical pain. And, we should recall, even pain is not just a fact. It is an *experience*, and, thereby, it is negotiated within a complex sensorial and *relational* matrix. We know, for instance, how the perception of labour pain widely varies depending on the ongoing emotional state of a woman; we are also aware of how a woman in labour benefits from a warm, sharing environment, where she can let herself go in her sensuous animality. She can then trust and abandon herself to the rhythm of her contractions, with no disturbing presence or messages, lights, or noises that might distract her from this magic moment of surrender to the impulsiveness of the baby who pushes to get out. A secure environment prevents the common enough complication that a woman, subconsciously, might, instead of opening up to help the child out, contract and hold him longer, without knowing that her body is really trying to protect her creature from an outside perceived as unfriendly. There is here an animal instinct that we must deal with, if only we could keep in mind that we, ultimately, are mammals, and "splendid" ones at that (Odent, 1999). Our survival-enhancing visceral preparedness, however, is negotiated, at the human level, within the actual conditions determined by one's emotional history and culture, both past and present; it is, therefore, liable to be distorted by what has passed before, evoked by similar contexts that trigger learnt responses which can haunt and hinder the natural template of expression of the instinct. For instance, by insinuating the freezing response led by an experience-based doubt that it is not safe to trust and let go (and, thereby, one should not ever do so again).

In my long experience, only twice have I agreed to a request for a C-section; both women had recently and tragically lost a child by violent death, and, emotionally, letting a baby out on his own still felt too much like a hopeless abandonment.

Therefore, I dislike the ease and superficiality with which these topics are usually treated, just as I think it unfair not to thoroughly inform the women of the risks associated with a C-section, or of the increase in operative deliveries following epidural anaesthesia. But my worries mainly regard something else.

What is close to my heart is defending the philosophical and emotional meaning of natural birth so that it may not be erased from awareness altogether, as if it were only a useless hyper-structure to an otherwise simply mechanical separation. During the already active analogic dialogue between an expectant mother and her child, even a momentary interruption of this link is clearly recorded, as it is between a mother and her newborn. I do not know, and cannot demonstrate, to what extent this might be harmful in every single case, but I am certainly worried not only about the effects on the baby during and after delivery, but also about the long-term consequences of a general indisposition to support an amount of effort, exertion, or endure patience beyond a certain threshold. In life, it is not always possible to turn to anaesthetics to deal with pain or the feeling, sometimes desperate, of not being able to cope. Besides, pain and joy, exertion and success, fear and solidarity, solitude and sharing, trepidation and waiting, all seem to me absolutely indispensable components of our existence; though sometimes painful and tragic, these are things that make our lives clearly fascinating, beautiful, passionate, intense, and absorbing. (Mieli, 2003, p. 39, translated for this edition)

Sanitised childbirths seem, therefore, to exemplify a more gener-alised difficulty in measuring ourselves against our feelings. Moreover, the medical profession's apparent keenness to avoid a woman's suffer-ing look to me more like a desire to mask the emotional complexity of the event and prevent a "threatening" expression and release of that naturally creative female power that a woman experiences and owns at the moment of childbirth.

> So it seems to me that there is an underlying, hidden weariness driving a need to put a gag on this female empowerment from the very begin-ning; a collective, unspoken wish to eliminate not only the disturbing emotionality of the woman giving birth, but also, and above all, the provocative, bursting, sensual, competent feminine corporeity that, in childbirth, boundlessly exudes a passion considered scandalous. Corporeity and feminine sensuality are the foundations of desire and feeling. The "feminine" epitomises the way of life that puts feeling before thought, not to exclude it, but to inspire it. Instead, a very differ-ent image of woman prevails: interchangeable in the erasure of differ-ences, aseptic, inflated, rubbery, easy to manage, and devoid of any complex feeling or ability to think or decide from the standpoint of her feminine reasonability. In other words, this is an image perfect for the kind of man who, save for rare exceptions, has long lost any physical and emotional connotation with what is truly masculine. Too insecure to trust his ability to elicit the desire of a woman, he resorts to control-ling her, reduced to a doll-like object. This ideal surrogate of woman is enticed with promises of discounts—literal ones, or from the effort of living—provided she accepts giving up her power, her competence at feeling and at making sense. And then, if she consents, in a world with-out feelings, she is offered the ease of interposing an early buffer between herself and her child, following a logic that will serve as a model for later, abrupt and aseptic separations to quicken and impose emancipation; exactly the opposite of what we know to be the basis, the foundation of the possibility for growth and for a true emotional acquisition of autonomy. (Mieli, 2003, p. 37)

I am still convinced of these bitter considerations when I think about the current model of femininity, which fluctuates between the anorexic model—walking broomsticks, taken as models of beauty by our adolescents, fearful to grow into women—and the abundantly remade, siliconised television showgirls. Both manageable surrogates of real feminine sensuality: as if to say that curves and features are acceptable only on a fake feminine, a low maintenance one, with which one can play and be entertained. While real women, outside the mould of fiction, are best deprived of any emotional aspect or sensuality that might champion the cause of feelings and needs, or disrupt the pragmatic flow of performativity.

Sexuality and motherhood in a woman are two strongly correlated aspects. There is a connection implied between physical areas and hormones, but, above all, there is a willingness to open up and receive, a giving and abandoning of oneself that facilitates and accompanies both functions. Research done by a midwife colleague of mine shows that women who are happy and uninhibited sexually—in other words, emotionally mature—give birth more easily. It also appears that providing women with a pre-birth training in affectivity during pregnancy fosters easier deliveries. The record holders in this small-scale research were my own patients, whom I worked with during their pregnancies for one affective disorder or another. They were looked upon as risky by my doctor colleagues because, in their opinion, to be referred to a psychotherapist one must be a "nutcase"— as they were elegantly classified among the staff—but eventually marvelled at by them all as, to everyone's surprise, my clients usually gave birth with the greatest of ease. This is because they were emotionally ready when the time came, having had the chance to attend to, understand, and appreciate their own emotional bio-feedback, recontextualised thanks to a reappropriation of their history.

I would, therefore, like to see the crucial nature of the emotional working-through that sustains and characterises pregnancy and childbirth returned to users. Given the times we live in, this, however, requires not only to extend the knowledge of affectivity and its workings to maternity ward staff, but also to the parents themselves, the protagonists, with their baby, in this story. This is to guarantee the possibility of a caring provision capable of grasping and appreciating the emotional aspects that are present in the doctor–patient relationship which currently go mostly unnoticed. I advocate a model of assistance able instead to pick up on affective communications, give them meaning, and support them. This approach to maternity care can perform an important role of prevention with respect to the pregnancy itself, facilitating its physiological progress up to delivery and post-delivery. Moreover, at the same time, it uses the entire process of maternity to pass on the simple embodied experience of the relational modalities that foster a developmental process. This can be invaluable in knowing the attitude to make one's own as a parent fostering the child's education.

It is often lamented that presently the know-how is no longer passed on from older to younger generations. Regarding discipline, this might be for the best because, even though the permissiveness that followed the 1968 student protests is creating serious problems, the authoritarianism that preceded it was certainly no less harmful. Even psychology, as we have seen, has only recently achieved a different, more balanced approach between containment and expression, acceptance and limits, security and freedom. So the matter seems to be not about transmitting old practices, but about having the courage to embrace a new framework, whose gist has been embodied in our own bio-psychological make up for us to read and discover, and to pass it on. Simply spreading this truth seems to me an inescapable ethical obligation.

I have practised from this standpoint for years with extraordinary results. Whenever I am given the chance, I still do, and when and where I am allowed, I always feel surrounded by great interest. I have always considered the role of a psychologist in the maternity ward up and foremost as a support to the staff, someone who works backstage in order to improve the quality of listening and, therefore, the entire service. I have tried to pass on to midwives the basic concepts of evolutionary psychology so they may then pass them on to pregnant women and couples, avoiding the need for too many "experts" in the maternity ward during childbirth preparation.

Sometimes, I am still invited to speak personally to parents awaiting the moment of delivery, introducing them to the physiology of the emotional unfolding taking place through pregnancy and in the development of a child's emotional world. I always feel deeply touched in witnessing the amazement and gratitude of some of these couples and mothers who, in their words, discover in my brief overview a way forward facing a vague and confused future, which is what parenthood looks like to so many expecting couples. Frequently, fathers react by saying: "I finally understand what the f*** I'm here for!". One father recently admitted, at the end of one of my lessons on affectivity, that he had just made two decisions: the first was regarding his possible presence in the delivery room, something I had made quite clear was not to be considered a duty, or a condition of being a good father—all of us having our own individual sensitivity that must be respected. He admitted to having had doubts, considering himself more of a hindrance than a help because of his own "emotional nature", but my affective and meaning-based description of the delivery convinced him he wanted to be the one to embrace his daughter as she came into the world, literally into his own hands. He would try. Second, when he came to the meeting he was unsure whether or not to accept a promotion at work. This would have meant a considerable increase in pay but also long periods of absence. He had made up his mind. He would turn down the offer because he was no longer willing to give up time he considered sacred, the time for being a father.

The real function of psychology in maternity

If the designated place for seeing a woman through to motherhood, whether it is a hospital or a doctor's office, were allowed to become contaminated with considerations regarding the emotions that come into play, then the woman being assisted would be reassured that her sudden emotional fits, her mood swings, and the whole ambivalence of pregnancy—with that distinctive mixture of joy about the process yet dismay or uncertainty about the novelty of the future ahead, inherently mixed with worries about her own adequacy as a future mother—are common emotional features: physiological aspects known to doctors and midwives and, therefore, perfectly admissible. Women would then know these emotions can be shared without shame. Therefore, an adequately attuned atmosphere, an awareness on the part of the staff in charge on how to treat, without fear, the emotional manifestations that come with pregnancy, would in itself be a preventative measure. Allowing and encouraging the free circulation and expression of emotions, in fact, would liberate them from reticence and shame, reducing the risk that something left unsaid today might be the cause of a difficulty or crisis tomorrow. In addition, given the right conditions, allowing for the free expression of emotional experience would make it easier to promptly identify—early detection being of the utmost importance for both physical and psychological disturbances in pregnancy—situations that show an unusual amount of anxiety or worries that go beyond the physiological flow of emotions that comes with any pregnancy.

Here is where I feel the psychotherapist's presence in first person is valuable in maternity, working alongside other staff members in detecting any early signs of a difficulty that should be noted and addressed. Psychotherapeutic working-through can then start from a legitimisation of the manifestation of distress—be it what it may—thanks to its contextualisation within the woman's life experience and attachment history. Then, taking advantage of the normative "regression" to childhood, the re-emergence and reparative holding of early traumas affecting the woman's capacity to trust—herself and the environment—makes it possible to embark on a journey of repair and transformation of patterns of relating, experiencing, and being. Pregnancy is thereby a most fertile moment, in my experience, for the suffering parts to be rehabilitated as valuable witnesses and allies in the building, thanks to the availability of support, of the woman's own mature capacity to love and care for the baby "as a real person, in his own right" (Guntrip, 1973, p. 385). It is as if pregnancy laid bare those voids everyone keeps hidden for fear of jeopardising their maturity. Instead, these voids need processing so that there may be trust and security.

Clinical referral must be delicate, avoiding anything liable to make it feel punitive or marginalising. It should, instead, be conveyed as an opportunity, naturally interwoven with standard care; an extra provision meant to help women arrive at delivery with a sense of tranquillity and emotional availability—a thousand times more useful for a newborn's physical and psychic health than all those obsessively repeated exams and check-ups. In the hyper-medicalised procedure of pregnancy assistance, the emotional bond linking mother and child, supported and facilitated by the serenity of the parental couple, is rarely taken into account, whereas this is the single most important factor ensuring a successful pregnancy, childbirth, and the child's future growth.

Sometimes, the experience of motherhood uncovers, as has been said, something unspoken, never admitted; something even less likely to be owned at this charged moment for fear of exhibiting a felt inadequacy at emotional coping, which the woman perceives as suddenly failing faced with the new test of motherhood. As we have said, the physiological ambivalence that accompanies pregnancy expresses itself in that mixture of feelings that keeps the woman suspended between fear and desire, between a dream and the fear of the novelty. This feeling is a healthy counterpart of a humble, yet accepting, attitude towards the task ahead; a stance mindful of one's own insecurities, but not overwhelmed by them. Ambivalence signals that a proper reflection on the ongoing change is taking place: attractive, but mysterious.

In cases where there is an unspoken distrust in one's emotional capacities, on the other hand, normative ambivalence appears instead "dramatised", tainted with an ancient distrust of oneself and the world. This weariness—disavowed and often never admitted or hidden behind a screen of success—is rekindled by the endeavour of motherhood and is invariably accompanied by intense fear and/or shame. For women who suddenly feel "invaded" by this sense of deep insecurity, it is like finding themselves face to face with something unforeseen, a neglected part of their self that suddenly turns up again.

From the therapeutic point of view, pregnancy is an exceptional period because of this very re-emergence of issues and difficulties that have been left unspoken, usually since childhood, and ever since kept in check through tight control, often unconscious. Pregnancy, moreover, is a time when we find an extraordinary accessibility to emotional experience, as if everything resurfaced at once and was there waiting for someone to finally hear it, understand it, and integrate what has hitherto never been processed. As explained in Chapter Two, this is due to the normative regression that stimulates in a woman a sensitivity very close to the one of her child, and, thereby, a re-emergence of feelings and emotions experienced in her own childhood in response to that particular way of perceiving the world. In light of this, working with a pregnant woman shortens the time of therapy. When I was working in a hospital, women had a voucher that allowed them eight appointments. That was enough for most of them. Others used two or even three vouchers—a limited time even so compared to standard therapy, precisely because of the great psychological availability connected with hormonal changes, as well as thanks to the strong motivation and determination linked to the desired creative process under way. I have always felt, and had many a concrete proof in feedback and in smoothness of delivery as well as security of attachment, that working therapeutically with these women accomplished a great task of prevention. Thanks to the sense of accompaniment throughout their pregnancy, these mothers could get to and through delivery and post-childbirth already accustomed to their emotions. Furthermore, having worked out their doubts and uncertainties through a shared reflection, they could experience a model of

attuned relatedness that could then be a tool in their own reper-
toires for them to facilitate free and healthy communication with their
children.

Identifying the difficulties and acting during pregnancy avoids having to deal with something more full-blown later on, which might lead
to more invasive interventions, and often when it is already too late.

I have always insisted my clinical work be "mixed" with the rest
of the activities in the ward, so that service-users could see an appointment with me as just another normal part of pre-childbirth care, helping those using the service not to feel singled out. Besides, if
psychological suffering, as we have seen, is linked to an early experience of inadequate care, what better chance can there be than during
pregnancy to revisit one's past and seek inspiration in experiencing a
new form of care and accompaniment? What could be better than
finally receiving help to understand and restore what went missing,
and thereby avoid any involuntary repetition of inadequate behaviour
toward one's own children? Motherhood is, or should be, an
emotional path for growth, a fertile period facilitating detachment
from, and reworking of, internalised models. This is a great opportunity for learning to be creative, emotionally too.

Sometimes, the difficulty of this passage is expressed through pain
and suffering a symptom. The range of psychic disorders that can arise
during pregnancy covers the entire spectrum of psychiatric events
and, as is well known in psychiatry, the nuances of emotional disorder
are infinite. This makes it almost impossible to catalogue and classify
them, as shown by the constant updating of the DSM (the American
Psychiatric Association's *Diagnostic and Statistical Manual of Mental
Disorders*, 1994), which is the most used diagnostic manual providing a
classification on the basis of descriptive clusters of symptoms.

Regardless of its fashionable popularity, it is, therefore, important
to stress that depression is not the only way a psychological disorder
can be expressed in pregnancy, and not necessarily only after delivery.
I underline this because, in the currently rampant psychiatricisation of
motherhood, depression is described and considered as almost
inevitable: a characteristic of motherhood to be monitored with a
battery of tests and controlled with psychotropic drugs. Hardly
anyone asks why on earth would nature want to inflict a woman, right
after childbirth, depression? What possible evolutionary value would
it have? A physiological post-partum depression (PPD) would, rather,

appear as something that would be conspiring *against* the survival of the species instead of working for its protection. Fewer still wonder at the growing frequency of this disorder and whether or not its occurrence might not instead be the result of long-neglected and repressed personal experiences in women's histories—often left unheard and unaddressed throughout their whole lives and even during pregnancy, given the generalised attempt to turn it into a purely medical procedure. Nobody seems to wonder if the growth in the incidence of PPD might be determined by the prevalence of contextual social constraints such as isolation, solitude, the suspension of work—with subsequent loss of reference points and contacts—leaving women alone in measuring up one's maturity against the new task without the support of an "adult" identity, mainly centred—in our workaholic society—on one's professional and social role outside the family.

Actually, on closer scrutiny, behind all the emotional disorders of motherhood—however expressed, with whatever symptoms—I have always found histories of suffering and solitude; stories of neglected or unloved but sensitive little girls, who find themselves alone facing, in motherhood, a much desired adventure that, nonetheless, frightens them, because something deep inside tells them they are not ready to face it; little girls who were not able to be little girls, but had to grow up fast; little girls who, as they, in turn, become mothers, secretly yearn for the cuddles and attention they have never had; or, on the opposite end, children whose growth was denied, who were kept under selfish wraps by anxious parents who never let them go, and as adults are unable to deal with the difficulties of life. In both scenarios, these women suffered a deficit in their own child-rearing, something very common given the past and present disinformation regarding the real emotional needs of childhood.

Therefore, in my opinion, there is no point in launching campaigns to monitor these women, rounding them up like rabid dogs to be isolated. To efficiently prevent perinatal psychological suffering, all it would take is structuring the existing care differently, so that women with a difficult attachment history would be able to voice their unease earlier and have an opportunity to experientially learn how to manage their feelings, for their own benefit as well as for their children's emotional future.

As has been said, lurking behind this feeling of inadequacy there is always a history of loneliness, of neglect of emotional needs, be it the one for attachment and/or the one for autonomy. Therapists know full well how children prefer to see themselves as bad rather than admit to being alone or mistreated, thus justifying the deprivation they suffer rather than revealing deficiencies in their parents. Maintaining the relationship is in fact vital, as without mum and dad there is actually no chance for survival for a little child. By taking upon oneself the responsibility for what makes one suffer, a child can fantasise that by changing herself—perhaps by being the good little girl—the situation will change for the better, keeping hope alive. If, alongside these wounds in a mother's own past, there is ongoing lone-liness, some conflict with her partner, or having to cope by herself with the fatigue that caring for an infant entails without external help or supporting relationships, then it becomes easy to understand how a woman might feel overwhelmed. Especially, if we also take into account that we live in a society that does little or nothing in favour of motherhood and appears exclusively bent on creating places where children can be parked so the mother can get back to work as soon as possible. Confronted by unfeasible motherhood models of perfection and self-sufficiency, it becomes easy to understand how a vulnerable woman might feel ashamed of being incapable, or less efficient than the system requires; she may lose heart and feel guilty, not because there is some intrinsic fault in herself—as she might well believe—but because human physical and emotional rhythms cannot keep up with those forced upon us by a society completely deaf to attachment needs.

A widespread attention to affectivity could, therefore, prevent many psychological disorders (perinatal as well as in the child) by identifying unresolvedness early, thus protecting the mother–child relationship during pregnancy and after birth. I am certain that even in terms of expenditure, this would be a much more convenient solu-tion than having to provide assistance to already dramatic situations that often require the attention of more than one specialist, if not dras-tic measures, such as hospitalisation, hardly compatible with a respect for the emotional needs of delicate moments such as pregnancy and childbirth.

* * *

Alongside all this, working daily in a maternity ward, I found another area where my services combined almost naturally with medical knowledge and assistance. I was frequently asked to intervene in cases where, unfortunately, the course of the pregnancy was disturbed by suffering and failure: spontaneous or involuntary miscarriages, interruptions due to foetal sickness, pregnancies where the foetus carried handicaps incompatible with survival, sudden stillbirths in the later stages of pregnancy or during delivery, the birth of severely premature infants and, more recently, assisted pregnancies in cases of infertility marked by numerous failures. Spending year after year with suffering couples, I learnt something really valuable that has enabled me to take a deeper look, and be able not just to bring comfort, but also interpret these stories of distress. I found that a search for meaning, even when facing such tragic events, helped my clients by inspiring and promoting awareness, psychological growth, and some valuable changes for future attempts at motherhood and, more generally, for life.

If we consider pregnancy as what it is, a crucial emotional event in the psychophysical development of women, and we accept it with its inherent ambivalence, common to all of life's significant passages, charged with wishful anticipation, yet also fear for the novelty of perspectives opening ahead, we can easily understand how a woman physically involved in this passage is at one with her emotional self. We can then understand how a potential *emotional* difficulty in trusting this project could lead, in the case of a vulnerable woman, to a *physical* lack of success. Therefore, I propose to consider the event in its indissoluble psycho-physical unity, where body and mind are considered inseparable and equally important components, each equally liable to bear a concrete influence. This also means that, even if the maternity care is open to listening and emotional expression, there are still women who, because of personal history or character, cannot allow themselves to show any existential uncertainty on an emotional level. In order to express such disavowed insecurities, it so happens that they might unwittingly resort to a somatic expression of their suffering, unconsciously perceived as being more acceptable and worthy of receiving attention.

The original mandate the hospital gave me was, in fact, much more formulaic and circumstantial: mourning should be handled by the psychologist. This is not always true, as I tried to demonstrate, training an emotionally prepared team. Referral to a psychotherapist does, however, become necessary when the pain does not abate, or when there is an inability to recover or restore meaning to one's life. Over years of practice, having held many a woman through a period of such deep mourning, I have discovered with them that, in these cases, the current pain always brought back some much older suffering. It was always as if the loss of the present echoed a string of other failures, adding a last ring in a chain of faults accompanied by a deep, nagging feeling of guilt and inadequacy. Or as if something, a deep personal truth, had been kept inside in solitude, with no chance to process it. Instead, the present mourning brought with it the unexpected opening of an encounter, a chance for sharing and a belated redemption. This, in turn, allowed putting a stop to an uncontrolled compulsion to repeat, linked to "not god enough" past relationships, to use Winnicott's term.

The present pain brought with it the opportunity to find empathetic care, the taste of a new and healthy relationship in the present that could nurture and saturate the voids left by past unmet needs. It was as if the bereavement had taken on the character of an extreme, desperate request from some repressed childhood part, wishing to be recognised and freed from the impossibility of expressing itself. I learnt in fact from clinical work that, when denied, these inner "little girls" never die, but remain as if frozen in time, still seeking a chance to be heard. They simply wait for some event, an unexpected failure, which could allow them to surface and make their voices heard in the desperate search for someone to meet their needs.

I discovered, for instance, how hyperemesis—a severe, persistent vomiting that can lead to serious weight loss during pregnancy—might hide an undeclared uncertainty about the event, often associated to a concrete situation of strain marked by solitude, financial constraints, relational problems, or separation from an emotional significant place or person. This, not surprisingly, is actually a common disorder among women from outside the European Union, who are more acutely aware during pregnancy of the weight and hardship of a long emotional separation. Hospitalisation is usually enough, and with it the implicit possibility of expressing a fragility that requires attention. Efficient care can entail anti-emetic treatments—which some colleagues sometimes exchange with placebos in order to test a possible psychosomatic origin—and, first and foremost, a relationship capable of holding and guiding through uncertainties and difficulties while confirming to these women their need for tenderness and protection as a normal feature of pregnancy. Any pregnant woman feels this way, and, therefore, it is paramount to convey a recognition of their need as legitimate, something that can be shared without shame, and comparable to what will be the experience and needs of the child. Just this provision normally ensures a significant amelioration, or even remission, whereas sometimes there is also a need for financial or social support. I remember a patient who had terminated her pregnancies due to hyper-emetic convulsions six times in a row, never having found a response capable of deciphering her suffering. I also treated a woman in her third pregnancy who had stopped eating and was sent to me with a nasal feeding tube that she stopped using after a few sessions. Here again, there was a legitimate reason behind her expression of pain, one tied to an experience of attachment insecurity going back a long way that was just waiting to finally be heard.

Miscarriages during the first three months of pregnancy are considered in the medical profession as almost physiological, due to the frequency with which they occur. As I have already mentioned, I all the same would rather society protected this trimester, and not the last one, with a suspension of work activity in order to support the need for rest that a woman suddenly perceives. Nature, in fact, by forcing her to slow down, intended to safeguard and strengthen the implantation of the egg in the uterus and the wondrous, incredibly complex and delicate process the foetus undergoes during the first trimester. Sometimes, miscarriages may occur several times—nine times for one patient of mine—or there may be a trail of oppressive suffering in need of clinical attention even after just the one. The medical team at the hospital where I worked had learnt to identify and distinguish the requests for help and send me only those whom they felt needed actual psychotherapy, rather than just a need to feel reassured and held, which they learnt with me how to happily provide themselves. Where referral was needed instead, I invariably found myself facing a situation of great insecurity in attachment and emotional regulation, worsened not only by the recent failure, but founded on a history of significant personal suffering. This compounded a deep sense of inadequacy, an anxiety towards life, an often disavowed as shameful fear of measuring up against reality: feelings that the woman herself feared ill suited to bear the weight of childbirth. Having someone to share the sense of responsibility, a secure relationship in which to process the bereavement and be supported through a new pregnancy—sometimes with a little supportive hormone treatment—has, in my experience, led not only to successful procreation but also to a general emotional maturation, and a happier life experience.

Sometimes, after successfully passing the fateful third month, some of these clients with a previous history of miscarriages would frantically land in my office and anxiously ask, apparently without reason, to interrupt the pregnancy. What causes this only apparently paradoxical behaviour is that, suddenly facing the prospect of success and no longer under the threat of a persistent fatality to which they could attribute the responsibility for failure, these women find themselves abruptly forced to face their own repressed fears and uncertainties. This unleashes such a massive dread as to convince them to want to renounce their plans. At other times, with the progress of the pregnancy, some of these women would start showing signs of disorders, sometimes severe behavioural disturbances that never occurred before, which required psychiatric help. These affective disorders, which I believe played an influential role in earlier failures, could then, thanks to the expression and meeting of a long denied need to be cared for, finally be addressed and overcome.

An even more complex clinical picture is found in cases of stillbirth—the death of the baby in the womb, at a late stage of pregnancy, or during labour. Bereavement here is even harder to cope with, when the mother has already enjoyed the pleasure of pregnancy, the perception of the baby's presence through his movements and signals, day and night. A loss like this is severe. The only way to overcome it, in my experience, lies in giving value to the baby's life, though short, and to the loving project that had sustained it, which will live beyond the failure. Naturally, this requires the ability to consider life in its entirety, including the value and reality of fantasies, hopes, and dreams. This value includes pre-life, a special time when a limited but significant relationship already exists between a mother and her baby, a relationship that the baby has been able to enjoy even in its brief existence. It is of great comfort to a mother to acknowledge and preserve the experience and meaning of the reality of this contact, of this early relatedness. It is important to celebrate its value, and cheer the bereaved mother's capacity and availability to provide a nurturing and caring containment. The abrupt interruption, and loss, seems in these cases to embody the actualisation of a terror, a feeling of abandonment in approaching the threshold of separation, the chill of becoming two persons. Stillbirths, in my clinical experience, are linked to complex past emotional experiences, the bereavement for the loss of a child echoing similarly tragic past events that were never fully processed. Spurred by the present intensity of the pain, profound absences and tragic losses suddenly resurface and facilitate a call for help, finally voicing a long-repressed need to be heard, and for a care expressed in a way that can soothe the pain. Working-through is about learning how to take, receive, and feel, recognising the right to feel loved—the only way to strengthen and consolidate the certainty of being able to give love. "I was a girl who fully trusted grown-ups. They suddenly threw me into a hell of guilt without much explanation. I didn't scream because I lost my voice and then . . . the repository for pain was already full. Everything is coming out now . . . this is really tough." These are the words of one of my patients, whose son died just before being born.

The resurgence of these disavowed childhood parts, finally heard and shared, and their integration, fosters, in my clinical experience, an extraordinary emotional growth in women and couples, an actual spiritual rebirth. This, in turn, facilitates the success of future preg-nancies—clearly also supported by medical treatment when necessary (even if unfortunately not always resolutive). I have met women who have lost three children in a row after the thirtieth week of pregnancy. Providing emotional support seems the least a public service could do for someone who has suffered so much, but efficacy is strongly depen-dent on the quality of the support provided. In my experience, it needs to be a provision of dynamic holding and guiding that is able to confront not only what is present, but also what has been carried over from the past. Only this in fact turns the therapeutic work from being only a soothing provision into an opportunity for emotional growth. My medical colleagues over time came to understand this well, as they regularly involved me in their treatments, feeling more protected when they shared with me their hopes and anxieties. I remember with particular fondness one of them who is no longer with us, Fabrizio, apparently the most sceptical of them all. "For me, women exist only from the waist down", he defiantly stated on our first encounter when I was trying to explain my presence to the medical staff on the maternity ward. I did not let his contrariness upset me, and from then on I took advantage of every break to chat with him and bring my message home—a sort of real seduction! Over time, Fabrizio became an admirer of my approach, and we shared many a clinical case that he wisely referred to me.

It is important in fact to remember that not only the women need emotional support in cases of mournful loss; it is important also to set up group supervision on the ward, providing a space to manage the anxiety of the medical staff after a tragic episode such as a recent still-birth. Only in this way, in fact, is it possible to contain the temptation of intervening too early on future occasions, out of fear or trying to magically avoid the date or period of the past fatal event. This, I am afraid, otherwise happens routinely, even if there are no scientific grounds to justify bringing forward the due date. Collective holding, instead, facilitates an attitude of respect of the unique schedule of any woman and child coming to the service. In cases of previous loss, this conveys a trust, albeit prudent, in the fact that something has changed thanks to the correct management and processing of the past bereavement.

* * *

I have often wondered, together with some of my most unfortunate patients, what distinguished their emotional paths from those of the many other women who are seemingly spared from having to face painful emotional ordeals and to work through their history before they can become mothers. Some women, in fact, have babies with the greatest of ease, although, politically incorrect as it may be to say, evidently unfit for the role of mother. I think the answer lies in the fact that, being unaware of any problem in themselves, these are women who have no ambivalence; they simply ignore any unresolvedness, so that nothing inside them stands in the way of their endeavour. For instance, I have worked with and seen a number of women—among whom were serious psychiatric cases—give birth with no trouble despite the misgivings of the specialists who treated them. I came to understand was that, by being overtly problematic, there was no real need for them to somatise their condition, which was not specifically linked to their pregnant state, because they already expressed it openly. Those who were instead more prone to psychosomatic manifestations were the most sensitive women, or women who, while appearing perfectly capable and efficient, were not inclined to "sentimentality", as they often put it. However, this second category of women prone to somatising harboured a secret weakness linked to their personal history—almost a preconscious premonition about the pregnancy—about which they dared not speak, since they did not know how to get out of this and did not want to be seen as weak. I have, therefore, come to think that the various ways and degrees a physical–emotional disorder is shown depend on the degree of denial, that is, how near or far from one's awareness is the knowledge of one's difficulty. Obviously, it is much harder to assist someone whose balance is the result of a long struggle to contain and repress her feelings, because this means acting on a lifetime of practice now firmly established. A personality has been built, for better or worse, upon a repressive habit which often not even pregnancy, with its hormonal imbalances, seems able to shift.

* * *

One of the most difficult losses to overcome for a woman is a therapeutic abortion; that is, when a pregnancy is terminated because of a congenital defect or illness of the unborn child. This is also due to the fact that, in most cases, the abortion takes place between the fifteenth and the twentieth week. By then, a mother has already felt the clear presence of her baby and, because performing curettage is no longer possible, actual childbirth must be performed by artificial induction. To avoid this sort of situation, mothers are increasingly advised to identify potential disabilities with early exams that may involve higher risk, though less so today thanks to more refined techniques. However, in this somewhat delirious race, spurred on by both medicine and service users, aimed at the elimination of whatever risk towards fulfilling a generalised sense of entitlement to see every wish guaranteed success, there is a huge omission. People still seem to forget, in fact, that even if it might look easier to intervene early, this, nonetheless, cannot cloak the earlier loss, still in need of being processed. From studies and comparisons of mothers mourning the loss of their child from voluntary interruptions of pregnancy and therapeutic abortions, there appears to be a dramatic difference between a renunciation, however difficult it may be, and a choice based on a child's disability. The first is usually connected with an assessment of reality, whereby the overriding preoccupation is not being in the proper emotional or material condition to receive a newborn baby and guarantee the care the child deserves; in the second case, instead, emotionally the interruption registers as if the baby were "discarded" as inadequate, casting somewhat of a shadow of inadequacy on the woman's capacity for maternal love too, which is unconditional by definition. It is very hard to do it without guilt; it is hard to give up a dream because of an unimagined difficulty for which one feels unprepared, unwilling, or insufficiently capable. Again, this is a painful admission of a limit, personal and situational. A lot of women find the strength and determination to give up when facing this limit and often their resolution is strengthened by worries about the difficulties a disabled child would encounter in a society already hardly suitable for "normal" children, let alone those who are not able to be self-sufficient. Naturally, this has nothing to do with the whims of those who only want ironclad pregnancies, and trouble-free, perfect babies, and who can always find compliant medical assistance for the right price. However, in my experience, even behind the fatality of a therapeutic abortion there can lie a lot more than fate. To an attentive ear, bereavement appears surrounded by a much broader emotional history. Here again, stories emerge of exertion, difficulty, and pain. I was recently deeply moved by the words of a young woman, frantic after a recent therapeutic abortion of her unborn child who had been diagnosed with a handicap incompatible with survival. At the end of an interview where details came out about a difficult and unaddressed personal history, she said to me, "I think I know why my child was not able to come into the world . . . I can't ask a baby to solve my problems with his presence . . . First, I must solve them myself in order then to be able to welcome a child."

* * *

I have frequently been involved in the births of severely premature babies. I am not referring here to cases of children recovered or treated for lack of development or insufficient amniotic fluid; the evolution of these cases, in fact, whether positive or negative, is generally more predictable, although parents would certainly benefit from greater emotional support, given the pain and precariousness of these conditions. I am instead referring to those abrupt, unexpected events when urgent action is required to save the child and sometimes even the mother. In these cases, in fact, the sudden, unforeseen prematurity often confronts the mother and couple with an extremely small newborn, sometimes less than 500 grams, the baby's survival chances uncertain and health conditions unstable, even though current medical and technological progress allows results that were unthinkable just a few years ago. Interestingly enough, it is within neonatal intensive care units (NICUs) that an attitude of greater sensitivity towards the emotional needs of neonates first appeared, a long time before any such consideration arose towards full-term babies. It is as if the increased observation and practice with these tremendously needy little beings had had the effect of finally convincing the world of children's "fragility mixed with strength", and of their need for the right kind of environment to survive. It is in NICUs that it was first realised how fundamental it is to encourage a rekindling of the mother–child bond as early as possible, so that she may guarantee the perception that the child has not lost the welcoming womb where he was formed. There must be greater attention to emotional aspects in NICUs.

Given the early separation—which, in itself, as we have seen, is always complex even in its physiology—in prematurity, however, the sudden interruption of an incomplete symbiosis, still in the making and transforming, is even more clearly evident. Yet, it has not been long that the medical profession has become aware of the baby's capacity to feel pain and of the analgesic effects of the maternal presence. Only recently, in fact, the idea has taken hold that these delicate creatures should not be exposed to intense lighting, or that they require some form of containment that may give them the illusion of the lost presence. If a baby born after the regular nine-month period still needs about three more months to realise that his mother is something external to himself as she relates to her in order to attend to his needs, then how much more difficult this passage from a "state" to a relationship must be for a premature baby who has yet to develop the cognitive means to perform such an operation? The practice called "kangaroo care" was devised to address these concerns. The naked baby is placed in direct contact, skin to skin, with the mother's or father's breast. The infant's biometrics are instantly enhanced, proving how important it is to re-establish symbiosis, since the warmth of his parents' human body is the baby's only known point of reference, recognisable by taste, contact, body heat, and sound and tone of voice.

When facing this unexpected event, mothers are obviously stunned and feel the weight of a failure for which they inevitably feel responsible, even though they might not be. Often, this sudden turn of events occurs in easy, happy, problem-free pregnancies and among women who remain active while expecting, when nothing leads them to believe there could be such trouble ahead. I know quite well the state of shock, disbelief, and anxiety that attacks those who experience the ordeal of a seriously preterm birth. This is a tragic event with an uncertain outcome. Many times, I have intervened in support of these anguished and desperate mothers, oppressed by deep feelings of guilt, asked to do all they can to assist the little baby fighting for his life. Obviously, support is required for the mother to get by, to continue hoping and get through the endless days of uncertainty, sustaining their trust and hope of not being a useless, helpless presence by their baby's side. Again, however, I found I could not, since the very first case referred to me—one I remember as if it were yesterday—limit my intervention to just a sympathetic ear. A young mother was fighting for her little girl, Annina, who weighed a mere 470 grams. She was desperate and when I met her she confessed to feeling the same desperation and helplessness as she did when she took her A-levels, which, in Italy, were at the time significantly called "Exams of Maturity". She told me how she had been terrified of being discovered not "mature enough". She spoke of herself, not of her baby girl. She was the one in need of support to become mature, so that she could be with her baby. She needed to be supported and contained, in order to then be able to contain in turn. The little girl came through and her mother got an unexpected opportunity in her life: to be offered a chance to retrieve and reintegrate a bit of her own history by expressing ancient disavowed needs.

Jean-Pierre Relier, a French paediatrician and neonatologist with, interestingly enough, a background in classical studies, after years of experience as director of neonatology at the Port Royal hospital in Paris, realised how important it is, when dealing with preterm infants, to assess the mother's emotional profile (see also Odent, 1986). Relier has written two illuminating books: *L'aimer avant qu'il naisse* (1993), an adequately eloquent title, and, in collaboration with Julia Pinchbeck, *Adrien ou la colère des bébés* (2002), which tells the story of a preterm baby and his mother and how he managed to save the baby, but also how the mother was supported by turning to less traditional methods, such as the services of an osteopath and even an astrologer.

In my own experience, too, the psychological profile of women at risk of preterm births is very specific. If it is true, as I believe, that difficulties in pregnancy go hand in hand with a woman's reluctance to admit her own fragility which instead is made more tangible by the event, I thereby came to believe that the power and extent of this denial is directly correlated to the differences between emotional configurations associated with problematic pregnancies, deliveries, or post-partum. For instance, what is surprising about unexpected preterm births is the ease of the pregnancy, almost as if the woman were unaware of being pregnant. Indeed, some women continue to have their periods as if they were not. Among these women, a somewhat ostentatious display of well-being, reported verbally as well as being apparent in behaviour and in an extremely self-confident, matter-of-fact demeanour, is not affected by the new state of expecting. In my team, I taught my colleagues to beware of these apparently easy patients who seemed to relieve them of any request for treatment or attention. The irreparable often happens unexpectedly.

I had identified some emotional signs, which I called "emotional markers", that singled out the pregnancies that stood out as "too easy", often showed off as uni-dimensionally happy events: late suspension of menstruation, hyper-efficiency, lack of any trouble, claims that they never felt so well, and long hours at work right up to the end. These markers helped to identify patients at risk and pay greater attention to situations that could evolve negatively. It would have been interesting to compare these women's personal and obstetric histories to have significant data on which to base my hypothesis. In fact, I came to observe how, in these cases of unexpected, extreme prematurity, the baby born so small and "unfit for life" appeared to be the image of a hidden child part of the mother's, equally felt as "unfit for life", to be repressed at all costs. These little-girl dissociated selves were awakened by the pregnancy but kept at bay by massive defensive measures. If and when these defences fell, the irreparable occurred. Working clinically with these women, I therefore had to guide them in retracing their personal histories and in how to take care of themselves first, in order to be able to look after their children later. The psychological struggle in these cases was not only for the survival of their offspring, but also for the affirmation of a part of themselves that had been neglected and denied until then. Understanding this allowed our team to approach mothers in the NICUs with greater consideration and an awareness that they could not work effectively on their own in supporting their child if no one was there to support them first; they had to be allowed to express their own, sometimes extreme, fragility and weakness in order to learn to love and accept it in themselves first, to then be able to meet that of the child's. It is important, as well, for the staff to be mindful that parents in these intensive care units, being there often for months, tend to learn the technical language and model the gestures used by the professionals. This is understandable, given the role of technology in keeping their children alive. But it is even more important for the staff to guide them to communicate physically and viscerally with their babies without fearing for their tiny size, dangerous only if deprived of an adequate emotional containment.

Only an affectionate and trusting view of her own fragility can allow a mother not to feel overwhelmed by the fragility of her child, so that she may not fall into the false seduction of trying to solve the unresolved dilemma between her adult and child parts through willpower and technology. This would, in fact, ultimately leave the needy aspects still devoid of affection and recognition.

*   *   *

Finally, working in a maternity ward, the impression is that the past ten years have seen an explosive rise of infertility. From a psychological standpoint, I can see that such a phenomenon cannot be explained without positing a shift in the somatic expression of psychological disorders associated with the emotional demands of pregnancy. This does not surprise me, since unresolved psychological dilemmas have taken on different forms of expression throughout history and changes in culture and customs. Undoubtedly, what we feel and how we feel is necessarily affected by the culture of the times in which we live. In Freud's time, when the social condition of women was quite different, the most widespread disorder was hysteria. Today, we see eating disorders being the most common, followed by depression. Cultural trends that sanction and dictate women's shapes and sizes certainly have great responsibility in the subconscious choice of a symptom. For those not strong enough to resist this influence, picking the body as the battleground against emotional needs felt as "too much", or as the expressive stage of feelings of inadequacy for a young woman desperately seeking a sense of social approval or success, makes sense if we think of how much more attention is bestowed on body shape rather than emotionality in our current day and age. Depression, as well as a form of communicative forfeit, is imbued with a sense of inability to express oneself or to be adequately recognised. Among women, in my opinion, depression also sanctions a sense of failure to live up to cultural norms that expect women to conform to a prevailing masculine model of efficacy. Legitimately, having been excluded from power for so long, women have desperately aspired to be "part of the game" with claims of dignity and equality. However, I believe the philosophical mistake hiding in the shadow of the feminist movement has been an insufficient focus on recognising, cultivating, and loving the specific strength and identity of our gender—irreducible to male values yet potentially capable of complementing them—as well as a failure to express this feminine identity with adequate persistence.

Assisted pregnancy programmes, however, appear not to be the least bit concerned about the emotional aspect that could lie at the basis of some issues of medically unexplained infertility; nor, they seem aware of the possibly serious consequences for a woman and a couple of numerous failures and of having to repeatedly face the prospect of their dream never coming true. I have often had the feeling of a cruel game being meticulously played on a purely physical and technical level, accompanied by a denial of any emotional connotation from either patients or staff. Clearly, in women torn by their frustrated desire for the realisation of a crucial aspect of their selves such as their reproductive creativity, the process can entail a progressive aggravation in their request. This can get to the point of becoming an obsession even, which, in turn, can make them willing to offer to do whatever it takes, accompanied as they understandably are by a growing feeling of anger and helplessness with each failed attempt. I have worked with a number of women who had repeated failed attempts at IVF, and I have always found, behind their desperation and insistence—yet again—histories of hidden, complex emotions kept at bay and sometimes denied. I am also aware that the truth is that their apparently entitled request to be equal to everyone else in terms of potential and self-fulfilment constitutes a claim for compensation due to unaddressed issues of deprivation. Paradoxically however, this same emotional denial exposes these women to some often frankly sadistic treatments. I have heard straight from their mouths the humiliation of being likened, because of their slight plumpness, to Scottish sheep that apparently ovulate less when overweight. I have witnessed their desolation when they submit to tiring monitored hormonal pumping, and when they are told how visibly dry and infertile their ovaries looked in the ultrasound scan. It is as if the medic were saying: "Look, I'm doing my best here, but if things do not work out, it's your own fault". The sanitised and unnerving procedure of assisted fertilisation, therefore, seems to me the current new expression of a desperate appeal for emotional attention, for a validation of adequacy as human beings with all their fragilities and never-met neediness, which instead continues to be denied through these retraumatising procedures.

We have come to such a point of denial that I have seen many couples who requested IVF without ever having had a sex life and sometimes never even wanting one. In their minds, there was no contradiction between wanting a baby and a relational life where the pleasures and power of intimacy were forgone. Having a baby was, for them, only the accomplishment of a project, the achievement of status, just like marriage; an only outwardly grown-up container that had never had to deal with the necessities of adult emotional life. Sadly, in these instances, technology is currently more than willing to offer a shortcut, even emotionally, to avoid any contact with feelings or with addressing a need for relatedness. The news is that instead, difficult to manage as it might seem to people who have never had the privilege of a secure attachment in childhood, a capacity for related-ness, secure dependency, and emotions remain essential for under-standing and caring for a baby.

However concerning this might be for the well-being of the child to come, nevertheless, technical and medical aspects seem to be the only issues at play in the awareness of both service users and staff when evaluating IVF. I have often responded to situations where women were desperate after several unsuccessful attempts, physically exhausted because of the intensity of the hormone treatments and the repeated emotional stress, often endured in complete solitude. Com-pounding the emotional strain, these women invariably harboured an obsessive belief that they were guilty of some unconquerable basic fault. These clients, in my experience, are some of the most demand-ing ones to hold. When there is infertility without medical reason, I have found that the repression of one's personal experiences was always very profound, hidden behind an usually extremely high level of efficiency. Ambivalence around willingness to change life habits to welcome a child into this world is also quite marked, but profoundly disavowed. A typical development, strange as it may seem to the layman, is the occurring of an unexpected pregnancy immediately following the decision to adopt: in other words, when the obstinate persistence for a successful fertilisation has been placated a little. As soon as the couple gradually begins to come to terms with their own limitations, without anger or shame, and starts to believe in their own ability and capacity for dedication to a creature whose presence in the world they were not directly responsible for, then conception magically happens.

Among unfertile couples, as I said, I have always encountered difficult life histories, great childhood suffering, either never or poorly processed, tales of emotional dependence suddenly cut off by a premature growth, often to relieve aggrieved parents; a growth, however, that was only mental and created by willpower. Such a developmental history understandably leaves the person, now an adult but only in name, with a strong resistance towards retracing the painful emotional course of her own existence. These situations usually developed, through therapy, into eventually successful pregnancies that were either spontaneous or assisted. In certain cases, the project was instead abandoned, as if, through therapy, these couples could come to accept their limit with a calm renunciation, with an easier and less regretful mind, almost a silent choice of a destiny more attuned to their own thwarted emotional needs, which now they could attend to.

CHAPTER SIX

Conclusions

I t seems to me that concerns regarding the devastating effects of a
social organisation with little or no awareness of, or respect for,
the importance of emotional life—and the necessity for it to be
protected and facilitated to allow everyone the acquisition of
emotional maturity—should be reinforced by the awareness of the fact
that this lack of attention not only has an impact on the mental health
of individuals, but can and will affect the mechanisms of our repro-
duction and survival as a species. The lower birth rate in our society
may already be ascribed to the challenging nature of current material
living conditions: the necessities of work, the pressure of financial
independence, and a general insecurity. However, in my experience,
low birth rates should also and increasingly be ascribed to more or
less explicit emotional difficulties that eat away at our trust in any
reproductive endeavour. If we do not take adequate care of our children, we will have unhappy and insecure adults (Brazelton &
Greenspan, 2001; Spitz & Cobliner, 1965). Society seems to be able to
respond to this concerningly common weariness by technological
prosthetics for childbirth, eliminating suffering, or making it possible
to have children artificially. But prosthetic technology fails to answer
many questions: it never helps growth, and it colludes in hiding the

insecurities that lay behind the difficulties and leaves them unmet, masking them with an apparent success. What has been missing—being heard, time, passion, and dedication—will continue to be missed, since no one understood that these things are what was needed in the first place. Suffering is, thereby, hidden instead of becoming understood and met, the only real instrument for change.

I believe that the evolution of society and an increased sensibility will eventually force us to face up to the extent of the damage done by inadequate emotional care. This societal progress in sensitivity shall, sooner or later, also convince us that only by guaranteeing a thought-through respect for emotional needs will it be possible to create a future in which procreation can be able to represent the plea-sure of passing life on to offspring together with that quality of love that alone makes our existence fascinating, enjoyable, and precious. This means guaranteeing, on the one hand, a general awareness of how our emotional world comes to grow. And consequently validat-ing and protecting the presence, assistance, and dedication to one's children on the part of both parents, facilitated in this by societal measures valuing and facilitating time spent with children.

To foster this I feel we need to spread awareness of the most powerful party's emotional responsibility towards the recipient of care in all nurturing or mentoring relationships and at all levels of society, covering all roles. This awareness should inform teachers, the various professions, commercial exchanges, even politics, so that living may come back to its relationality: a joint effort that should include every-one in fostering emotional willingness and cooperation; namely, those very social characteristics natural selection appears to have chosen long ago as guarantees for maintaining and improving human exis-tence.

But, for this to come to pass, this awareness must be known and word must be spread. Otherwise, there can be no change, because all of this can happen only through a conscious collaborative effort. Again, this is a matter of riding nature "taoistically", so as to under-stand it and give it full expression. I have never considered a healthy emotional life to be incompatible with a safe, solid, economic organi-sation—quite the contrary. But an economic organisation, in order to be sustainable, cannot base itself on the denial of material needs (disparity of rights has already sparked many a revolution), just as it cannot thrive without safeguarding emotional needs. Expanding an attitude of consideration and respect for these needs would inevitably bring changes in our way of living, probably healthy ones if we consider the current scenario. Fewer things, fewer goods, and more relationships could be a good motto if only we all finally understood that the human need for relationships is not an option that can be denied. Relationships are the natural emotional–biological condition that make the survival of our species possible and, as such, can no longer be neglected and ignored.

*   *   *

As for me, I have worked with this model of care applied to pregnancy for over twenty years in two different hospitals and have described my experiences and successes in numerous conferences and discussion panels. I have enjoyed the esteem of my colleagues, the passionate interest of many new parents, and the affection of women and couples whom I was able to help, despite having absolutely insufficient working hours compared to the time required in this field of work.

This wonderful experience ended with the retirement of the enlightened chief of maternity who made it all possible with his passion and far-sightedness.

My hope, in writing this, is to reach a sensitive and intelligent readership that may make use of my reflections so as to share a new outlook on life and offer inspiration. Expert or laymen, parents, teachers, or health workers, encouraging each and every one of us to gain a new awareness and a concern that may lead our society to a greater respect for the emotional–relational sphere of existence. This, in my view, would be necessary in both our work environments and in our everyday life. Human life requires the restoration of an openness and coherence attainable only by striving for that healthy combination of feminine and masculine I have tried to convey and give justice to in this book, in the description of conception, pregnancy, childcare, and emotional growth. This matrix alone can guarantee, along with happy relationships with others, little ones and grown-ups, that inner well-being and serene enjoyment of existence we all aspire to: a promise made in our very psycho-emotional potential, which needs our consciousness, both individual and collective, to be realised.

BIBLIOGRAPHY

Ainsworth, M. D. S., Blehar, M. C., Waters, E., & Wall, S. N. (2015). *Patterns of Attachment: A Psychological Study of the Strange Situation*. Hove: Psychology Press.

Benasayag, M., & Schmit, G. (2003). *Les passions tristes. Souffrance psychique et crise sociale*. Paris: La Découverte.

Bernal, J. D. (1965). *Science in History*. London: Penguin.

Bestetti, G., & Regalia, A. (Eds.) (2007). *Il dolore è... nel parto*. Milan: Mimesis.

Bowlby, J. (1951). *Maternal Care and Mental Health (Vol. 2)*. Geneva: World Health Organization.

Bowlby, J. (1969). *Attachment and Loss: Attachment*. New York: Basic Books.

Bowlby, J. (2005). *A Secure Base: Clinical Applications of Attachment Theory*. New York: Routledge.

Bowlby, J., & Ainsworth, M. D. S. (1965). *Child Care and the Growth of Love*. London: Penguin.

Braibanti, L. (1993). *Parto e nascita senza violenza*. Novara: RED.

Capra, F. (1997). *The Web of Life: A New Scientific Understanding of Living Systems*. New York: Anchor Books.

Capra, F. (2004). *The Hidden Connections: A Science for Sustainable Living*. New York: Anchor Books.

Cavallari, G. (2001). *L'uomo post-patriarcale*. Milan: Vivarium.

Cavalletti, G. (2003). *Laura: storia di una bambina piccolissima e della sua voglia di vivere.* Venice: Marsilio.

Centro Italiano Psicologia Analitica (CIPA) (2002). *Il padre. Parola, silenzio, trasformazione – Atti dell'XI Convegno nazionale, CIPA.* Milan: Vivarium.

Cigoli, V., & Scabini, E. (2007). *Family Identity: Ties, Symbols, and Transitions.* London: Routledge.

Damasio, A. R. (1999). *The Feeling of What Happens: Body and Emotion in the Making of Consciousness.* San Diego, CA: Harcourt.

De Duve, C. (2002). *Life Evolving: Molecules, Mind, and Meaning.* Oxford: Oxford University Press.

Décant-Paoli, D. (2002). *L'haptonomie.* Paris: PUF.

Edelman, G. M. (1992). *Bright Air, Brilliant Fire: On the Matter of the Mind.* New York: Basic Books.

Edelman, G. M. (2006). *Second Nature: Brain Science and Human Knowledge.* New Haven, CT: Yale University Press.

Einstein, A. (2015). *Relativity: The Special and the General Theory.* Princeton, NJ: Princeton University Press.

Fava Vizziello, G., Zorzi, C., & Bottos, M. (1992). *Figli delle macchine.* Milan: Masson.

Foot, P. (2003). *Natural Goodness.* Oxford: Clarendon Press.

Freud, S. (1974). *The Standard Edition of the Complete Psychological Works of Sigmund Freud.* London: Hogarth Press.

Galimberti, U. (1979). *Psichiatria e fenomenologia.* Milan: Feltrinelli.

Galimberti, U. (1999). *Psiche e techné.* Milan: Feltrinelli.

Gamow, G. (1985). *Thirty Years that Shook Physics: The Story of Quantum Theory.* North Chelmsford, MA: Courier.

Giddens, A. (2011). *Runaway World: How Globalisation is Reshaping Our Lives.* London: Profile Books.

Greenspan, S. I., & Benderly, B. L. (1997). *The Growth of the Mind and the Endangered Origins of Intelligence.* New York: Perseus Books.

Grotstein, J. S., & Rinsley, D. B. (1994). *Fairbairn and the Origins of Object Relations.* New York: Guilford Press.

Guntrip, H. (1973). *Personality Structure and Human Interaction,* J. D. Sutherland (Ed.). London: Hogarth Press.

Husserl, E. (2013). *Cartesian Meditations: An Introduction to Phenomenology.* Berlin: Springer Science & Business Media.

Infeld, L. (1971). *The Evolution of Physics.* Cambridge: Cambridge University Press.

Jung, C. G. (1954). *The Collected Works of C. G. Jung.* Princeton, NJ: Princeton University Press.

Klein, M. (1975). *The Psychoanalysis of Children*, A. Strachey (Trans.). Oxford: Delacorte Press/Seymour Lawrence.

Klein, M. (2017). *The Collected Works of Melanie Klein*. London: Karnac.

Kohut, H. (2009). *The Restoration of the Self*. Chicago, IL: University of Chicago Press.

Kuhn, T. S. (1970). *The Structure of Scientific Revolutions*. Chicago, IL: University of Chicago Press.

Latouche, S. (2007). *Petit traité de la décroissance sereine*. Paris: Mille et une nuits.

Lim, R. (2001). *After the Baby's Birth: A Complete Guide for Postpartum Women*. New York: Henry Holt.

Lorenz, K. (1974). *Civilized Man's Eight Deadly Sins*, M. Latzke (Trans.). London: Methuen.

Mancia, M. (1998). *Coscienza sogno memoria*. Rome: Borla.

Marinopoulos, S. (2005). *Dans l'intime des mères*. Paris: Fayard.

Miller, A. (2008). *The Drama of the Gifted Child: The Search for the True Self*. New York: Basic Books.

Nagel, E. (1961). *The Structure of Science: Problems in the Logic of Scientific Explanation*. San Diego: Harcourt, Brace & World.

Naranjo, C. (2009). *L'ego patriarcale*. Milan: Urra.

Naranjo, C. (2016). *Changing Education to Change the World: A New Vision of Schooling*. Newburyport, MA: Hampton Roads.

Paci, E. (1973*). Idee per una enciclopedia fenomenologica*. Milan: Bompiani.

Relier, J. P., & Pinchbeck, J. (2002). *Adrien ou la colère des bébés*. Paris: Laffont.

Rizzolatti, G., & Sinigaglia, C. (2008). *Mirrors in the Brain: How Our Minds Share Actions and Emotions*. Oxford: Oxford University Press.

Shiva, V. (2005). *Earth Democracy; Justice, Sustainability, and Peace*. Brooklyn, NY: South End Press.

Stiglitz, J. E. (2007). *Making Globalization Work*. London: W. W. Norton.

Tomasello, M. (2008). *Origins of Human Communication*. Cambridge, MA: MIT Press.

Vallino, D. (2005). *Raccontami una storia*. Rome: Borla.

Vallino, D., & Macciò, M. (2006). *Essere neonati*. Rome: Borla.

Watts, A. (2017). *Psychotherapy East & West*. Novato, CA: New World Library.

Winnicott, D. W. (1998). *Thinking about Children*. Boston, MA: Da Capo Press.

REFERENCES

American Psychiatric Association (1994). *Diagnostic and Statistical Manual of Mental Disorders: DSM-IV.* Washington, DC: American Psychiatric Association.

Balint, M. (1955). The doctor, his patient, and the illness. *Lancet, 265*(6866): 683–688.

Bellieni, C. V. (2004). *L'alba dell' "io". Dolore, desideri, sogno, memoria del feto.* Florence: SEF.

Bertirotti, A. (2008). *Un'interpretazione cognitiva dell'etica. Scienza e società.* Milan: Università Bocconi.

Bertirotti, A. (2009). *L'anima cerebrale.* Acireale-Rome: Bonanno.

Bertirotti, A., & Larosa, A. (2005). *Umanità abissale.* Acireale-Rome: Bonanno.

Bowlby, J. (1944). Forty-four juvenile thieves: their characters and home-life. *The International Journal of Psycho-analysis, 25*: 19.

Bowlby, J. (1988). *A Secure Base. Parent–Child Attachment and Healthy Human Development.* New York: Basic Books.

Bowlby, J. (2012). *The Making and Breaking of Affectional Bonds.* New York: Routledge.

Brazelton, T. B., & Greenspan, S. I. (2001). *The Irreducible Needs of Children: What Every Child Must Have to Grow, Learn, and Flourish.* Boston, MA: Da Capo Press.

Brazleton, T. B., & Sparrow, J. (1992). *Touchpoints: Birth to Three*. Boston, MA: Da Capo Press.

Brazelton, T. B., & Sparrow, J. (2008). *Touchpoints: Three to Six*. Boston, MA: Da Capo Press.

Capra, F. (1984). *The Turning Point: Science, Society, and the Rising Culture*. New York: Bantam.

Capra, F. (2010). *The Tao of Physics: An Exploration of the Parallels Between Modern Physics and Eastern Mysticism*. Boston, MA: Shambhala.

Chiarelli, B. (1997). Evoluzione del cervello e nascita dell'autocoscienza. *Sistema Naturae*, 4: 19–34.

Chiarelli, B. (2003). *Dalla natura alla cultura. Principi di antropologia biologica e culturale*. Padua: Piccin.

Damasio, A. R. (2008). *Descartes' Error: Emotion, Reason, and the Human Brain*. London: Random House.

De Waal, F. B. (1996). *Good Natured: The Origins of Right and Wrong in Humans and Other Animals*. Cambridge, MA: Harvard University Press.

Deutsch, H. (1945). *The Psychology of Women (Volume 2). Motherhood*. Oxford: Grune & Stratton.

DiBlasio, P., & Ionio, C. (2001). Elaborazione emotive e sintomatologia da stress post partum. *Psicologia della salute*, 2: 27–45.

Dolto, C. (1999). *L'haptonomie périnatale*. Paris: Gallimard.

Estivill, E., & Anderson, R. (2008). *5 Days to a Perfect Night's Sleep for Your Child: The Secrets to Making Bedtime a Dream*. New York: Ballantine.

Estivill, E., & Domènech, M. (2005). *Si mangia!* Milan: Feltrinelli.

Fairbairn, W. R. D. (1957). Freud, the psychoanalytical method and mental health. *British Journal of Medical Psychology*, 30(2): 53–62.

Fairbairn, W. R. D. (1994). *Psychoanalytic Studies of the Personality*. New York: Routledge.

Ferenczi, S. (1968). *Thalassa: A Theory of Genitality*. New York: Norton.

Ferliga, P. (2005). *Il segno del padre*. Bergamo: Moretti e Vitali.

Fornari, F. (1976). *Simbolo e codice*. Milan: Feltrinelli.

Fornari, F. (1977). *Il Minotauro*. Milan: Rizzoli.

Fornari, F. (1981). *Il codice vivente*. Turin: Boringhieri.

Freud, S. (1930a). *Civilization and its Discontents*. S. E., 21: 59–145. London: Hogarth.

Fried, E. (1991). Was es ist [What It Is] in *Love Poems*, S. Hood (Trans.). New York: Calder.

Gallese, V. (2007). Before and below 'theory of mind': embodied simulation and the neural correlates of social cognition. *Philosophical Transactions of the Royal Society B: Biological Sciences*, 362(1480): 659–669.

Gallese, V., & Lakoff, G. (2005). The brain's concepts: The role of the sensory-motor system in conceptual knowledge. *Cognitive Neuropsychology*, 22(3–4): 455–479.

Gallese, V., & Umiltà, M. A. (2002). From self-modeling to the self model: agency and the representation of the self: Commentary by Vittorio Gallese and Maria Alessandra Umiltà. *Neuropsychoanalysis*, 4(1): 35–40.

Gaskin, I. M. (2003). *Ina May's Guide to Childbirth*. New York: Bantam Dell.

Gerhardt, S. (2004). *Why Love Matters. How Affection Shapes a Baby's Brain*. Hove: Brunner-Routledge.

Giordana, M. T., Fava, C., & Zappelli, M. (2001). *I cento passi*. Milan: Feltrinelli.

Goldstein, J. (1999). Emergence as a construct: history and issues. *Emergence*, 1(1): 49–72.

Guntrip, H. (1973). *Personality Structure and Human Interaction*, J. D. Sutherland (Ed.). London: Hogarth Press.

Heisenberg, W. (1958). *Physics and Philosophy: The Revolution in Modern Science*. New York: Prometheus Books.

Herbinet, E., & Busnel, M. C. (1981). L'aube des sens. *Les cahiers du nouveau-né*, 5: 4–211.

Honegger Fresco, G. (2006). *Facciamo la nanna*. Turin: Il Leone Verde.

Husserl, E. (1954). *Husserliana, Band VI, Die Krisis der europäischen Wissenschaften und die transzendentale Phänomenologie*. The Hague: Martinus Nijhoff.

Husserl, E. (1970). *The Crisis of European Sciences and Transcendental Phenomenology: An Introduction to Phenomenological Philosophy*. Evanston, IL: Northwestern University Press.

Jones, E. (1953). *The Life and Work of Sigmund Freud*. Oxford: Basic Books.

Jones, E. (1994). Preface. In: W. R. D. Fairbairn, *Psychoanalytic Studies of the Personality* (pp. v–viii). New York: Routledge.

Juul, J. (2001). *Your Competent Child: Toward New Basic Values for the Family*. London: Macmillan.

La Repubblica (2007). Interview with D. Morris, author of *La scimmia nuda*. 4 April.

Laing, R. D. (1982). *The Voice of Experience*. London: Allen Lane.

Laing, R. D. (1990). *The Politics of Experience and the Bird of Paradise*. London: Penguin.

Latouche, S. (2004). *Survivre au développement: De la décolonisation de l'imaginaire économique à la construction d'une société alternative*. Paris: Fayard/Mille et une nuits.

Lorenz, K. (2002). *King Solomon's Ring: New Light on Animal Ways*. Hove: Psychology Press.

MacLean, P. D. (1972). Cerebral evolution and emotional processes. *Annals of the New York Academy of Sciences, 193*: 137–149.

Maggioni, C., Margola, D., & Filippi, F. (2009). PTSD, risk factors, and expectations among women having a baby: a two-wave longitudinal study. *Journal of Psychosomatic Obstetrics & Gynecology, 27*(2): 81–90.

Mahler, A., & Pine, F., & Bergman, A. (1975). *The Psychological Birth of the Human Infant: Symbiosis and Individuation.* New York: Basic Books.

Marcus, G. (2004). *The Birth of the Mind: How a Tiny Number of Genes Creates the Complexities of Human Thought.* New York: Basic Books.

Mieli, G. (2003). *La presenza dello psicologo nei reparti di Ostetrica e Ginecologia. Perché? La psicologia nelle Aziende Ospedaliere e negli IRCCS in Lombardia.* Turin: Centro Scientifico Editore.

Miller, A. (1990). *Thou Shalt Not Be Aware: Society's Betrayal of the Child.* New York: Farrar, Straus and Giroux.

Miller, A. (1997). *Breaking Down the Wall of Silence: The Liberating Experience of Facing Painful Truth.* London: Penguin.

Miller, A. (2002). *For Your Own Good: Hidden Cruelty in Child-rearing and the Roots of Violence.* New York: Farrar, Straus and Giroux.

Miller, A. (2006). *The Body Never Lies: The Lingering Effects of Cruel Parenting.* London: W. W. Norton.

Miller, A. (2012). *Banished Knowledge: Facing Childhood Injuries.* London: Virago.

Morin, E. (1992). From the concept of system to the paradigm of complexity. *Journal of Social and Evolutionary Systems, 15*(4): 371–385.

Morin, E. (2013). *La méthode: la nature de la nature.* Paris: Le Seuil.

Naranjo, C., & Houston, J. (2010). *Healing Civilization.* Oakland, CA: Rose Press.

Nathanielsz, P. W. (1992). *Life Before Birth and a Time To Be Born.* Ithaca, NY: Promethean Press.

Needham, J. (1925). *Science, Religion and Reality.* London: Sheldon.

Needham, J. (1929). *The Sceptical Biologist.* London: Chatto & Windus.

Needham, J. (1931). *The Great Amphibian.* London: SCM.

Needham, J. (1936). The biological basis of sociology. In: *Time: The Refreshing River (Essays and Addresses, 1932–1942).* New York: The Macmillan Company, 1943.

Needham, J. (1945). *Time, the Refreshing River.* London: Sheldon.

Needham, J. (1958). *Science and Civilization in China.* Cambridge: Cambridge University Press [reprinted Cambridge: Cambridge University Press, 1965 and 1973].

Needham, J. (1968). *Order and Life.* Cambridge, MA: MIT.

Needham, J. (1969). *The Grand Titration*. Crows Nest, Australia: Allen & Unwin [reprinted Abingdon, 2013].

Neruda, P. (2003). Cierto cansancio [A certain weariness]. In: *Estravagario* (Volume 367). Barcelona: Debolsillo (translated for this edition).

Odent, M. (1980). *Human Birth: For an Ecological Change in Childbirth*. Munich: Koesel Verlag.

Odent, M. (1986). *Primal Health*. London: Century Hutchinson.

Odent, M. (1988). From psychoendocrinology to primal health. In: P. Fedor-Freibergh & P. Vogel (Eds.), *Prenatal and Perinatal Psychology* (pp. 439–448). Lancs, UK: The Parthenon.

Odent, M. (1999). *The Scientification of Love*. London: Free Association.

Paci, E. (1965). *Relazioni e significati*. Milan: Lampugnani Nigri.

Paci, E. (1970). *Funzione delle scienze e signifcato dell'uomo*. Milan: Il Saggiatore.

Pallante, M. (2005). *La decrescita felice*. Rome: Riuniti.

Paul VI (1967). *Encyclical Letter. Populorum progressio*. Available at http://w2.vatican.va/content/paul-vi/en/encyclicals/documents/hf_p-vi_enc_26031967_populorum.html

Phillips, A. (1988). *Winnicott*. London: Fontana.

Phillips, A. (1999). *Saying" No": Why It's Important for You and Your Child*. London: Faber and Faber.

Pietropolli Charmet, G. (Ed.) (1987). *La democrazia degli affetti*. Milan: Cortina.

Rapisardi, G. (2005). *Le mani con il neonato ... cosa sappiamo. Mani nel parto, mani sul parto*. Milan: Carrocci.

Relier, J.-P. (1993). *L'aimer avant qu'il naisse*. Paris: Laffont.

Relier, J.-P., & Pinchbeck, J. (2002). *Adrien ou la colère des bébés*. Paris: Laffont.

Righetti, P. L., & Sette, L. (2000). *Non c'è due senza tre*. Turin: Bollati Boringhieri.

Schmid, V. (1998). *Il dolore del parto*. Firenze: Centro Studi Il Marsupio.

Schmid, V. (2005). *Venire al mondo e dare alla luce*. Milan: Urra.

Schmid, V. (2007). *Salute e nascita*. Milan: Urra.

Schmid, V. (2011). *Birth Pain: Explaining Sensations, Exploring Possibilities: A Guide for Midwives*. Chester: Fresh Heart.

Schore, A. N. (1997). Early organization of the nonlinear right brain and development of a predisposition to psychiatric disorders. *Development and Psychopathology, 9*(4): 595–631.

Sen, A. (1987). *On Ethics and Economics*. New York: Basil Blackwell.

Sen, A. (1997). *Resources, Values, and Development*. Cambridge, MA: Harvard University Press.

Shiva, V. (1988). *Staying Alive: Women, Ecology and Survival in India*. New Delhi: Zed Press.

Siegel, D. J. (2012). *The Developing Mind: How Relationships and the Brain Interact to Shape Who We Are* (2nd edn). New York: Guilford Press.

Siegel, D. J., & Hartzell, M. (2003). *Parenting from the Inside Out: How a Deeper Self-understanding Can Help Raise Children Who Thrive*. London: Penguin, TarcherPerigee.

Spitz, R. A., & Cobliner, W. G. (1965). *The First Year of Life*. Madison, CT: International Universities Press.

Steiner, R. (1973). *Sigmund Freud e la psicoanalisi*. Naples: Morano.

Suttie, I. D. (2014). *The Origins of Love and Hate*. London: Routledge.

Teilhard de Chardin, P. (1957). *Le Milieu Divin*. London: Fontana.

Teilhard de Chardin, P. (2015). *The Phenomenon of Man*. Morrisville, NC: Lulu Press.

Tinbergen, N. (1951). *The Study of Instinct*. London: Oxford University Press.

Tomasello, M. (2009). *The Cultural Origins of Human Cognition*. Cambridge, MA: Harvard University Press.

Verny, T. R., Kelly, J., & Pennycook, R. (1981). *The Secret Life of the Unborn Child*. New York: Summit Books.

Volta, A. (2006). *Apgar 12*. Pavia: Bonomi.

Whitehead, A. N. (1967). *Adventures of Ideas*. New York: Free Press.

Whitehead, A. N. (1997). *Science and the Modern World*. New York: Free Press.

Whitehead, A. N. (2010). *Process and Reality*. New York: Simon and Schuster.

Winnicott, D. W. (1958). *Through Paediatrics to Psychoanalysis: Collected Papers*. London: Tavistock [reprinted London: Routledge, 2014].

Winnicott, D. W. (1964). *The Child, the Family, and the Outside World*. London: Penguin [reprinted London: Penguin, 2000].

Winnicott, D. W. (1965a). *The Family and Individual Development*. London: Tavistock [reprinted Abingdon, Oxon: Routledge, 2006].

Winnicott, D. W. (1965b). *Maturational Processes and the Facilitating Environment: Studies in the Theory of Emotional Development*. London: Hogarth Press.

Winnicott, D. W. (1971). *Playing and Reality*. London: Tavistock [reprinted London: Penguin, 1990].

Winnicott, D. W. (1988). *Human Nature*. London: Taylor & Francis.

Winnicott, D. W. (2014). *Through Paediatrics to Psycho-Analysis: Collected Papers*. London and New York: Routledge.

INDEX